Dr. Fischer's Little Book of
Big Medical Emergencies

DR. FISCHER'S LITTLE BOOK OF

BIG

Medical Emergencies

How to Recognize and Respond to the Most Common Medical Emergencies

Stuart Fischer, M.D.
Edited by Mark D. Steisel

BOOKS
Fort Lee • New Jersey

Published by Barricade Books Inc.
185 Bridge Plaza North Suite 308-A
Fort Lee, NJ 07024
www.barricadebooks.com

Illustrations by Susan Grisell

Library of Congress Cataloging-in-Publication Data
Fischer, Stuart.
    [Little book of big medical emergencies]
    Dr. Fischer's little book of big medical emergencies : how to recognize and respond to the most common medical emergencies / Stuart Fischer ; edited by Mark D. Steisel.
        p. cm.
    Includes index.
    ISBN 1-56980-241-6 (pbk.)
    1. Medical emergencies--Popular works. 2. Medical emergencies--Handbooks, manuals, etc. I. Steisel, Mark D. II. Title.

    RC87 .F5346 2002
    616.02'5--dc21

                                                                        2002026108

First Printing
Manufactured in Canada

Dedication

This book is dedicated to Dr. David Grob, the Director of Medical Education at Maimonides Medical Center during my medical student, internship, and Internal Medicine residency. I feel honored to have been taught by him, and to learn from his warm, caring, and always inquisitive approach to the art and science of practicing medicine.

—Dr. Stuart Fischer

To my wife, Sara Slavin, and my mother, Hedy Green, for their love and support.

—MDS

Contents

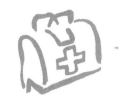

Contents

Contents

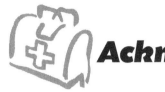 # **Acknowledgments**

My most grateful thanks go to the following people who contributed their time and expertise and helped make this book a reality. Dr. Bertrand Agus (internist, rheumatologist), Dr. Sigmund Chessid (orthopedist), Dr. Avram Cooperman (surgeon), Dr. Amy Glaser (pediatrician), Violet Kelly R.N. (the finest nurse I have ever worked with and an excellent teacher herself) and Susan Grisell, a prize-winning Impressionist artist who has stressed the relationship of man to nature, who contributed the illustrations. Her honored work has been exhibited in New England and New York City and her paintings are included in private collections throughout the world.

We wish to thank and express our enormous gratitude to all of those who have helped and supported us in making this book a reality. Thanks especially to Rick Frishman who brought us together and who has steadfastly been with us through this entire project.

Thanks also to Division Chief Brian Waterbury, San Rafael, CA Fire Department, Martha Meador, Gay Lynn Duel, Margo Rohrbacher, and Jeannie Huffman.

Introduction

At some point, you'll probably have to respond to a medical emergency. *HOW YOU RESPOND COULD SAVE YOUR LIFE OR SOMEONE ELSE'S.* When a medical emergency arises, will you:

• Know what to do?
• Know what not to do?
• Know how to give and/or get successful treatment?
• Be able to help save someone's life?

In medical emergencies, knowledge is critical. You don't have to go to medical school or even learn complicated terms and procedures. However, you should—at the very least—get a basic understanding of medical emergencies that could affect you, your friends, and loved ones. That is what this book provides.

Medical emergencies can range from superficial cuts and bruises to profound, life-threatening problems. Often, they're difficult to diagnose and distinguish. Medical emergencies affect not only patients, but families, friends, and those who witness these often horrifying events.

The purpose of *Dr. Fischer's Little Book of Big Medical Emergencies* is to help non-medical people respond quickly and effectively to emergencies. To achieve this purpose, it is written in the most clear, direct language, with a minimum of technical terms. All medical language has been clearly defined. This book has been designed to give readers easy access to vital information so they can act quickly and with confidence.

Introduction

This book includes:

- Basic instructions on giving emergency care
- An explanation of how the emergency care system works
- Instructions (with illustrations) on how to perform CPR, take a pulse, stop bleeding wounds, make a splint or tourniquet, and figure out if the patient is breathing normally
- An index of symptoms to quickly diagnose emergencies
- Chapters devoted to each of the most common medical emergencies, which explain:

    1. What each emergency is
    2. How to recognize it
    3. What to do
    4. What not to do
    5. What treatment to expect in the emergency room
    6. Typical follow-up care
    7. Comments by Dr. Stuart Fischer

Keep a copy of this book in your home, workplace, car, boat, and recreational vehicle. The information it contains could save a life!

Basic Principles of Emergency Care

1. Approach any emergency in a *calm* and *orderly* manner. When a patient is relaxed and confident, you increase the odds for a successful recovery. Diagnosis and treatment are easier and the patient is more likely to help—rather than hinder—caregivers. Conversely, an alarmed patient can impede those who are trying to help. If you are the caregiver, don't panic or show your fears. If you are the one having the medical emergency, remain as calm as possible.

2. Be observant; take inventory. Identify and assess the general nature of the problem. Is it an orthopedic, surgical, medical, or psychological emergency? Is the patient awake, responsive, and comfortable? Is the patient unconscious? Do you feel a pulse? Is the patient breathing (regardless of the reason why)? Are there any life-threatening injuries? Has the patient been removed from the source of danger?

3. If possible and if time permits, find out whether the patient has a preexisting medical condition and which prescription medication(s) he/she is taking. However, don't delay calling 911 while you are conducting a lengthy search of the patient's medicine chest.

4. Call 911. When in doubt, call 911 as soon as possible. It makes no sense to delay, guess, or take foolish chances when professional help is just a phone call away.

5. When you call 911, respond to the questions they ask. The information you provide may be vital in saving the patient's life. Don't guess. If you don't know an answer, say so. The operator will move on to the next question.

6. Ask the 911 operator what you can do until the emergency care technicians arrive. Write down all instructions in the order in which they should be carried out. The 911 operators are professionals who deal regularly with medical emergencies so make sure that you understand their instructions and follow them precisely. If you don't understand any instructions, ask for clarification.

7. Call friends and neighbors to assist or stay with you until emergency technicians arrive. Don't leave the patient unattended. If you don't feel up to the tasks at hand, get help.

8. When emergency care technicians arrive, let them do their job. Follow their instructions and assist them if they ask for your help. Don't ask questions or get in their way when they are providing emergency care. Be patient. Let the experts do their work. You will have a chance to ask questions after they have stabilized the patient.

9. Stay nearby. Be available to answer questions or to provide any assistance they request.

How Emergency Systems Work

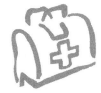

Emergency medical systems operate under a triage or priority system, which operates both before patients reach the hospital and upon arrival. Basically, here's how it works.

1. When 911 calls are received, dispatchers send highly trained emergency care technicians (ambulance and paramedic personnel) to the scene. The dispatchers question callers and send technicians to the most serious emergencies first. They also relay all information that you provide to the emergency technicians, often while you are still on the phone with them.

2. Upon arrival on the scene, the emergency care technicians evaluate the patient's condition. They may rely heavily on your observations. The technicians initiate treatment and decide whether and where to take the patient. When dealing with heart attacks, technicians may radio a physician who will direct them to give oxygen, an IV and morphine, nitroglycerin, or other medication. A patient suffering from multiple, life-threatening injuries may be rushed to a specialized trauma center rather than a general hospital.

3. Upon arrival at a medical facility, patients with the most serious conditions are seen first, their problems are diagnosed and treatments are started. Diagnostic testing usually includes obtaining the patient's history, a physical exam, Xrays, electrocardiogram, and blood tests. Some emergencies (hip fractures) may be immediately apparent, while others (aortic aneurysms) may be more elusive. When you go to an emergency room, the first person you will talk to is a triage nurse whose

duty it is to prioritize your medical problem. Triage is a concept first formulated on the battlefield where those individuals with the most severe treatable injuries needed to be attended to first. Because of the varied nature and enormous range of typical medical emergencies, your particular problem may not be dealt with immediately (cardiac and trauma patients always have priority), and you may need to wait to see a physician. Moreover, some emergencies need diagnostic tests to be performed (blood tests, Xrays) that will lengthen the time the patient will stay in the hospital.

4. Many conditions may take hours to precisely diagnose. Specialists may be required. So be prepared to wait. Bring warm, comfortable clothing, reading material, and lots of patience.

When You Call 911

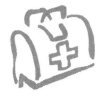

1. The first thing you hear will be, "911. What is your emergency?"

   - The 911 dispatcher is a highly trained professional who knows the right questions to ask and is there to help.
   - Tell the dispatcher if it is a medical emergency, a fire, a hazardous material spill, etc., if you know.
   - As briefly as possible, tell the dispatcher the victim's condition. For example, "My husband isn't breathing," "My son is bleeding profusely," "He won't wake up."
   - Briefly tell the dispatcher what happened. "He just fell in the kitchen." "He fell off a ladder." "She overdosed."
   - Get to the point. The more information the dispatcher gets quickly, the more it will help. While you are giving the information, the dispatcher may be relaying it to emergency workers.
   - Be calm and try not to panic. Your response could frighten the victim, which could worsen his condition, and make it difficult for the dispatcher to get important information.

2. Know the correct address. Although the dispatcher will know the address where the call was placed, you will be asked to verify the address where the emergency workers should go. This is necessary because you may be calling from a neighbor's house, from a public place, or on a cell phone.

   a. If you are calling from somewhere other than your home, know the address where the victim is.

b. If you are calling from a large public place, describe as precisely as possible where the victim is.

c. If you are in a large store, a mall, or a place with multiple entrances, ask someone who works there which entrance the emergency team should use.

d. If you are calling from a cell phone, know where you are and where the emergency team should go.

3. Remain on the phone until the dispatcher tells you to hang up. If you hear a click or silence on the other end, don't hang up. Assume that the dispatcher placed you on hold while emergency help is dispatched. Expect the dispatcher to get back on the line to ask you additional questions.

4. Let the dispatcher take command. Dispatchers are trained to deal with panicked callers. Some distressed callers can waste valuable time by being long-winded, impatient, argumentative, and even hostile. Keep calm, cool, and focused. Trust the dispatcher and pay attention!

5. Be prepared to answer follow-up questions including "Has this ever happened before?" "What caused the victim's fall?" "How far did he fall?" "What medication is he on?" Once the emergency workers are on their way, the dispatcher may ask you for further information and relay your answers to the emergency workers.

6. Follow the dispatcher's instructions. If the dispatcher tells you to perform a procedure, she will explain exactly what you should do, step-by-step. She may tell you how to apply direct pressure on a wound, perform CPR, or clear a blockage with the Heimlich maneuver.

7. Many 911 centers have multilingual capabilities. Dispatchers will find out what language you speak and instantly contact a translator who speaks your language and will join you in a three-way conversation.

Hospital Admission and Ability to Pay

A hospital that provides emergency care cannot reject, refuse to treat, or transfer patients because they cannot pay or do not have health insurance. Under the Emergency Medical Treatment and Active Labor Act (42 USC 395dd), commonly called the Federal Patient Anti-Dumping Act, a hospital is required to give a medical screening examination to all patients who arrive at its Emergency Room in order to rule out that they do not have a life threatening medical condition. Screening exams and required treatment cannot be delayed to inquire about the patient's financial status or ability to pay.

If the screening exam reveals that the patient has a medical emergency, the hospital must provide treatment within its capability to stabilize the patient's condition or transfer the patient to a facility with the requisite capability.

For example, if a pregnant woman who is in labor goes to the ER, the hospital must admit and treat her until the child is born and they can safely leave. However, if a patient with severe burns goes to a hospital that does not have a burn-care unit, the hospital will not be required to provide treatment because treating burn victims is beyond its capability. However, such hospitals will generally give emergency first aid care and transfer the patient to a facility that is equipped to treat burn victims. The facility that receives the patient will then be required to provide care within its capability regardless of the patient's financial status or ability to pay.

The Emergency Medical Treatment and Active Labor Act was enacted in 1986 to prevent hospitals from refusing to accept patients who could not pay (dumping). Previously, those rejected were forced to go or would be taken to charity and government-run hospitals, which were often further away. The law applies to all hospitals that receive federal funds, which includes virtually all U.S. hospitals with the notable exception of the Shriner's Hospitals for Crippled Children.

What is an Emergency?

The hospital staff will usually decide if an emergency medical condition exists. The law specifies that the patient must have symptoms of sufficient severity that if he/she does not receive immediate medical treatment, his/her health could reasonably be expected to be in serious jeopardy, incur serious impairment of bodily functions or serious dysfunction of any body part or organ. With respect to pregnant women who are having contractions, an emergency exists when there is inadequate time to safely transfer the patient to another facility before delivery or when the transfer might threaten the health of the mother and her unborn child.

Medical Emergencies

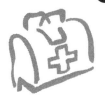

Abdominal Pain

What It Is

Although abdominal pain is often listed as the number one cause of Emergency Room visits, the complex anatomy of the digestive tract often makes it difficult to diagnose the precise cause of the pain. Abdominal pain may be due to one of more than twenty different illnesses or to trauma. Pain may come from a ruptured or inflamed organ or from irritation or inflammation of the inner lining of the abdominal cavity (the peritoneum). The causes of abdominal pain can be grouped into four anatomical categories:

- Gastrointestinal: appendicitis, gallstones, intestinal obstruction, pancreatitis, and diverticulitis.
- Genitourinary: kidney stones and urinary retention.
- Gynecologic: tubal (ectopic) pregnancy and pelvic inflammatory disease.
- Vascular: ballooning of the aortic (aneurysm), abdominal angina.

Some abdominal conditions pass quickly while others are chronic. Abdominal pain may come on gradually or suddenly. It may be continuous or intermittent and range from mild to excruciating. To complicate matters, abdominal pain may be of minor significance or life-threatening and the cause can be unrelated to its apparent location ("referred pain"—for example, feeling right shoulder pain during gallstone attacks). Conditions such as gallstones, bleeding ulcers, appendicitis, and kidney stones have several symptoms in common. Therefore, even mild and vague abdominal pain must be considered potentially significant.

Other causes of abdominal pain include small bowel obstruction (due to scarring from prior abdominal surgery), intestinal strangulation (a twisting of the intestines that cuts off the blood supply), pancreatitis (usually due to alcoholism or gallstones), diverticulitis (inflammation/infection of small pouches in the large intestine), and kidney disease (renal colic). Abdominal pain may also indicate cardiac disease since the lower portion of the heart shares nerve fibers with the upper gastrointestinal organs.

Gastrointestinal Bleeding

Bleeding may occur anywhere along the gastrointestinal tract; in the esophagus, the stomach (peptic ulcers, erosive gastritis), small intestine (duodenal ulcer), large intestine (fragile blood vessels in the colon, diverticulitis, or colon cancer), or the rectum (internal or external hemorrhoids). Virtually all patients with gastrointestinal bleeding will require hospitalization, but the treatment will vary according to each patient's condition and the amount of blood loss.

What To Look For

- Paleness, pain, rigidity, and severe tenderness over the entire abdomen may indicate **peritonitis, the most serious abdominal emergency**. Peritonitis results when an organ ruptures into the abdominal cavity, irritates the inner lining, and shuts off all gastrointestinal functions. The abdominal muscles become tight and severely painful to touch.
- Nausea, vomiting, diarrhea, or unstable blood pressure (manifested by dizziness, severe fatigue, or "feeling cold").
- Watery diarrhea, vomiting, and abdominal cramps, but no localized abdominal pain, tenderness, or signs of peritonitis (acute gastroenteritis caused by either a virus or salmonella).
- Abdominal pain in an elderly patient with severe arteriosclerosis, hypertension,

cold feet, and leg cramps when walking may indicate an aortic aneurysm. This is a major medical emergency. Call 911 at once.

- Abdominal pain, nausea, and vomiting that are triggered by exertion and relieved by rest (or nitroglycerin) can indicate a heart problem. Call 911 immediately.
- Sudden onset of abdominal pain in children or the elderly can be the sign of appendicitis. The pain may initially appear anywhere in the abdominal area, but it usually begins around the belly button and localizes in the lower right region after 24 hours.
- Rectal bleeding, black bowel movements, or vomiting blood or "coffee-ground" material (gastrointestinal bleeding).

What To Do

- Call 911 immediately when abdominal pain lasts more than a few minutes and the patient feels faint or turns pale.
- Call 911 immediately if an elderly patient with severe arteriosclerosis, hypertension, cold feet, and leg cramps has abdominal pain.
- Call 911 immediately if abdominal pain, nausea, and vomiting occur with exertion and are relieved by rest or nitroglycerin.
- Keep a patient who is not dizzy or pale seated and leaning slightly forward.
- Keep the patient relaxed and comfortable.

What Not To Do

- Don't attempt to diagnose or treat anything but the most minor gastrointestinal symptoms (such as heartburn occurring after big, rich, or spicy meals).
- Don't give a patient with potentially serious abdominal pain anything to eat or drink.
- Don't allow a patient to lie on his/her back because vomiting may occur. Instead, turn the patient to one side.

Typical Treatment

The ER staff will question the patient about the onset, nature, intensity, duration, and apparent location of the pain. The patient's vital signs will be taken and may reveal low blood pressure and a rapid heart rate, which suggest loss of fluid (pancreatitis) or hemorrhage (perforated ulcers). Intravenous fluids are immediately given to stabilize the patient's circulation. Physical examination of the abdomen may reveal the root of the problem and/or the existence of peritonitis. Blood tests, Xrays and other examinations (sonograms, CT scans, colonoscopy) will also be employed.

Laboratory and Xray tests are required to diagnose pancreatitis, gallstone attacks, and often appendicitis. All women of childbearing age will receive a pregnancy test to rule out tubal pregnancy, which accounts for many surgical emergencies.

Pain medication cannot be given until the cause of the pain is determined because it might mask the manifestations of an illness (or even peritonitis). Before a treatment plan is set, the patient's condition will be confirmed and reconfirmed by:

1. Reviewing the history of the illness
2. Physically examining the patient
3. Analyzing laboratory tests (blood, urine and Xray)

Specific treatment will vary depending on the condition diagnosed. Treatments might include: surgery for a ruptured spleen, intravenous fluids for kidney stones, antibiotics for diverticulitis, or all of the above for appendicitis.

The length of hospital confinement will depend on how quickly the patient was treated and if complications developed. It may range from several hours for a mild intestinal virus to several weeks for repair of an aortic aneurysm.

For gastrointestinal bleeding, a tube will be placed through the patient's nose to wash out the stomach. Since blood is an irritant, it must be removed from the gastrointestinal tract. Bleeding may be treated during an endoscopy, the procedure performed to inspect the inner walls of the esophagus, stomach, and large intestine. After severe gastrointestinal bleeding, the initial blood tests may be misleadingly normal.

Follow-up Care

A patient with abdominal pain will be hospitalized unless his/her symptoms resolve completely in a few hours. Even a patient who doesn't require hospitalization should be reevaluated within the next twenty-four hours.

The ER staff will determine whether a surgical consultation is warranted. A patient with a ruptured aortic aneurysm or appendicitis complicated by peritonitis may be rushed to surgery within an hour.

Some episodes of abdominal pain are of brief duration and of unknown origin. A patient diagnosed with "nonspecific abdominal pain" will be ordered to see his/her personal physician within twenty-four hours or to return to the ER if the symptoms persist or worsen.

Acute appendicitis may resolve if fecal material blocking the entrance to the appendix is dislodged and passed through the intestine.

Surgery complicated by peritonitis may require hospitalization for a month or longer.

Dr. Fischer Says

To examine the abdomen, gently push down about one-half inch and circle around the belly button. If the area feels as hard as wood and the patient is pale, suspect peritonitis and immediately call 911. Some facts: appendicitis is the number one cause of abdominal pain for patients under age fifty; gallstones are the primary cause of abdominal pain for those over fifty.

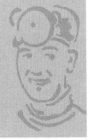

Appendicitis

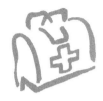

What It Is

The appendix is a tiny, fingerlike pouch that sits at the end of the small intestine to the right of the belly button. Although it has no known function, it can cause serious emergencies, usually in children and adolescents. Most cases of appendicitis (and diverticulitis) occur when hardened fragments of feces block the pocket's tiny opening and restrict the normal secretion of mucus into the intestine, causing the appendix to swell. Trapped bacteria flourish and attract cells from the immune system in nearby tissues. In worst-case situations, untreated swelling and infection can block the blood supply (causing gangrene) or rupture into the abdominal cavity (causing peritonitis), a life-threatening emergency.

High risk groups include children, pregnant women, and the elderly. Children under six have a high rate of perforation and peritonitis.

What To Look For

- WARNING: Whenever a child has abdominal pain, suspect acute appendicitis, no matter how slight, no matter what area seems to be affected. A running, playing, or eating child is unlikely to have appendicitis. However, a child who has pain when coughing may have peritoneal irritation.
- Initial mild discomfort in the center of the body around the belly button usually moving to the right lower abdomen over a four to forty-eight hour period.
- Pain in any area of the abdomen or even in the lower back. The symptoms for acute appendicitis can resemble many other disorders. For example, the pain and

discomfort may be mild and resemble heartburn. Elderly patients (or those taking steroids) may have more vague discomfort or no symptoms at all.
- Nausea, vomiting, and loss of appetite.
- Low-grade fever—especially in young children.
- Discomfort and immobility.

What To Do
- Call 911 immediately.
- Keep the patient immobile. Unnecessary movement could cause the appendix to rupture and send bacteria into the abdomen. When in doubt, always err on the side of caution and call 911. The problem could quickly become serious and most office-based physicians lack the proper equipment to diagnose this emergency.

What Not To Do
- Don't give the patient medication, painkillers, or other remedies. They could mask important symptoms.
- Don't touch or examine the patient. Touching could worsen the patient's pain.

Typical Treatment
Diagnosis of acute appendicitis is based on the progressive development and migration of the patient's pain. Acute appendicitis may resolve if the fecal material that blocked the entrance to the appendix is dislodged and passes through the intestine.

The potential for serious complications makes exploratory surgery the best treatment. Furthermore, standard tests can be misleading. When peritonitis is suspected, the appendix will be surgically removed without waiting for test results.

As a result, surgery is often performed on patients even though as many as twenty percent of them may not have appendicitis. When the diagnosis is less clear and the patient's condition seems less severe, sonograms or CT scans of the lower abdomen will be ordered. If they reveal an inflamed, enlarged appendix, the appendix will be surgically removed.

Uncomplicated appendicitis cases require only a few days hospitalization. However, when an appendix ruptures and bacteria spread into the abdomen, surgery becomes more involved. In addition to removing the ruptured organ, the entire area must be cleansed to prevent the formation of adhesions (scarring) and abscesses.

A postoperative patient may remain on intravenous antibiotics for several days or weeks depending on the severity of the condition. The patient is not allowed to eat for several days after surgery because the gastrointestinal tract shuts off and food cannot be properly digested until normal operation resumes.

Follow-up Care

Appendicitis usually requires little follow-up care. When surgery is performed, one or two office visits are needed to check on how the incision is healing.

A patient who is discharged from an emergency room with an unclear but suspicious diagnosis should see a physician within twelve to twenty-four hours. The patient should not take painkillers (including aspirin) or antibiotics unless authorized by the physician.

Dr. Fischer Says

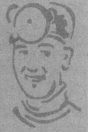

Six percent of us have had our appendix removed. Do you still have yours? Originally, the appendix was probably a mini-storage area that functioned like one of a cow's three stomachs to help with the digestion of grass. However, as the human diet changed over millions of years of evolution, the appendix became unnecessary. Unnecessary or not, it can still cause problems and severe pain.

*Back Injuries**

What They Are

Essentially, the spinal column is a stack of small bones (called vertebrae) that surrounds and protects a network of nerves. The nerves connect the brain to a vast system of receptors, muscles, and organs throughout the body. The vertebrae sit one atop another, supported by muscles and separated by discs (softer, elastic cushions that help us bend and rotate). An irritated or inflamed ligament, tendon, muscle, or bone in the lower back can generate intense pain. About eighty-five percent of the time, no definitive diagnosis or precise source of the back pain is found.

Some people are prone to back injuries because of inherent, inborn spinal weaknesses, but most injure their backs when they strain to lift heavy objects or lift objects in an awkward manner. These movements disrupt the spinal column's alignment and damage ligaments and tendons. Discs may slide out of position, compressing or irritating nerves; discs may also rupture and disc material may ooze out, compressing or irritating nerve roots. To prevent discs from slipping and causing further damage, the muscles in the area contract into a spasm. Although back spasms are painful, they prevent movements that could cause serious neurological damage.

Sciatica occurs when an injury to the lower spine irritates the nerve roots that form the sciatic nerve. This sends pain through the buttocks, down the back of the thigh, and down the leg on one side of the body, often as far as the toes. A patient typically feels lower back pain, "pins and needles" sensations, or numbness in one foot. The patient may also limp or favor one leg and/or find it uncomfortable to sit or stand.

*Cervical spine or neck injuries are discussed in a separate chapter entitled Neck Injuries.

Back Injuries

Spinal stenosis is a narrowing of the central spinal canal that is often mistaken for sciatica. As the cord compresses, it causes numbness in both legs that creates difficulty walking. Spinal stenosis is a degenerative condition that often accompanies osteoarthritis and is not due to physical injury. Sitting often helps to relieve the pain.

Fractured vertebrae can cause the spinal column to partially collapse. Spinal fractures are painful and are usually caused by osteoporosis (a gradual process of bone loss common in older women), injury, or cancer that has spread to the spinal column.

What To Look For

- Severe back pain, or "pins and needles" (tingling and numbness of the arms or legs). Pain may intensify with physical movement.
- Shooting pain down the buttocks and leg (sciatica) or in the shoulder and arm.

What To Do

- Most patients with back pain don't need to call 911.
- However, you should call 911 if pain:
  - Occurs suddenly.
  - Occurs immediately after strenuous physical exertion (or within twenty-four hours of it).
  - Is triggered by a cough or sneeze.
  - Is excruciating.

A doctor may not have the necessary office equipment to assess the condition and may refer the patient to an orthopedist or an emergency room. Most patients with lower back pain can sit in a car long enough to be driven for emergency treatment.

- Call 911 when any of the following neurological symptoms occur for the first time:
  - Tingling ("pins and needles").
  - Pain radiating down the leg.

- Numbness.
- Difficulty walking.
- Loss of bladder control.

What Not To Do

Don't move a patient who has sustained a back injury. Also, do not allow the patient to walk or move until healthcare professionals arrive. Movement can cause permanent neurological damage.

Typical Treatment

Since muscle spasms usually prevent disc slippage, most lower-back pain does not involve nerve compression. Therefore, treatment focuses on the spasms. Oral muscle relaxants such as Valium®, Robaxin®, or Flexeril® are prescribed as are anti-inflammatory medications including Motrin®, Indocin®, and Advil®.

Although Xrays of the affected area are usually taken, they only reveal bone damage such as fractures. Xrays don't show damage to nerves, discs, ligaments and tendons, or muscle spasms.

If nerve injury is suspected, a CT scan or MRI will be ordered to view the soft tissue between vertebrae. Patients will remain hospitalized only when emergency surgery is required.

Follow-up Care

Recovery and follow-up care depend on the severity of the condition and how quickly it was diagnosed and treated. Bed rest does not speed recovery from sciatica, but two or three days of bed rest on a firm mattress is still usually recommended.

Most patients are urged to resume their normal activities as soon as possible. They are given exercises to perform and instructions on proper lifting and bending techniques.

Chiropractors and acupuncturists can frequently relieve sudden back pains, but only if Xrays are negative and "slipped" (herniated) discs are not suspected. Many patients with chronic low back pain benefit from physical and rehabilitative therapy.

Dr. Fischer Says

When a patient has "pins and needles" sensations, call for emergency medical assistance immediately, especially if it was triggered by a cough or sneeze. Within two months of an injury, the condition of ninety to ninety-five percent of all patients will improve regardless of the type of treatment they receive.

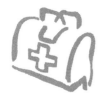

Bites

Animal Bites

What Are They?

Human, dog, cat and other animal bites account for one percent of all ER visits. Snake, spider, scorpion, and insect bites are discussed in this chapter. Marine creature bites are discussed on page 117.

Human bites can transmit life-threatening infections because the human mouth contains bacteria that flourishes in the absence of oxygen. Unrecognized infections can turn fatal after twelve hours. Human bites occur almost exclusively on the hands or arms from intentional bites or from punches that contact the teeth. Herpes and hepatitis B viruses can also be transmitted through bites.

Dog, cat, and other animal bites can puncture the skin, crush tissue and bones, cause infection, and transmit rabies. Although damage from most bites is superficial, serious injuries can occur that require immediate medical treatment. For example, a bite that just barely breaks the skin can still cause a serious infection. Infections emanate from bacteria in the animal's saliva. The likelihood of infection is influenced by the animal's size, the puncture's depth, and the patient's age. Children and the elderly are most prone to infections.

Cat bites occur far less frequently than dog bites. But cat bites, and cat scratches, can produce more infection than dog bites. Cats' sharp and thin teeth can penetrate deeply, injuring tendons, nerves, and blood vessels. These wounds are often hard to clean. Also, cats frequently lick their claws so even minor scratches can become easily infected.

Bites

What To Look For
With the Animal
- Foaming at the mouth, which indicates rabies.
- The type of animal involved. Bats, skunks, raccoons, and foxes are rabies transmitters.
- Whether the animal is wild, a stray, or a pet (pets generally have been vaccinated).

With the Patient
- Bleeding.
- Open puncture wounds, cuts, scratches, and scrapes.
- Swollen glands near the site of a cat scratch about one week after the scratch occured.

What To Do
- Find out what kind of animal inflicted the injury. This may make a difference in the type of treatment required.
- Call 911 immediately.
  - For human, skunk, raccoon, fox, and bat bites.
  - If the animal was foaming at the mouth, wild, or a stray.
  - If a wound is deep, open, or continues to bleed.
- Stop bleeding by applying gentle pressure on the wound with a clean cloth until the bleeding stops.
- Cleanse closed wounds with antiseptic soap or sterile water.
- Rush the patient to the nearest ER.

Typical Treatment
Human bites are never sutured because some bacteria from the human mouth thrive in the absence of oxygen. Wounds are cleansed and irrigated with fluids, explored (if severe, in an operating room), and kept elevated. Intravenous antibiotics are given.

Bites

Dog, cat, and other animal wounds are cleaned with antiseptic soap and sterile water. Large wounds will be sutured, but small wounds will usually be left open, irrigated, and covered with sterile dressing. A patient will receive tetanus toxoid injections if he/she has not been immunized in the past five years. The patient will also be evaluated to see if minor surgery and/or antibiotics are needed. A cat bite victim is usually given antibiotics because cat bites are hard to clean.

When rabies is suspected (in skunk, bat, raccoon, and fox bites), a patient is given immunoglobulin and booster vaccines.

Follow-up Care

Wounds usually close without the need for suturing. They should be examined every two to three days to monitor the healing process and check for infection.

A red streak leading away from the wound may indicate bacteria traveling through the tissues. This is a sign that intravenous antibiotics are needed.

Dr. Fischer Says

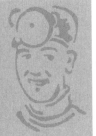

Each year in the U.S., dogs are responsible for several million reported bites. Patients who were bitten by humans, however, are frequently too embarrassed to seek medical attention even though they may need it more than those attacked by animals. Make sure all human bite victims get prompt medical attention because they may not show signs of infection until twenty-four hours after they were injured.

Snake Bites

What They Are

Snakes usually attack only when disturbed. Their bites are dangerous because they may inject poisonous venom into their victims through their long, sharp fangs. Venom from pit vipers (rattlesnakes, water moccasins, and copperheads) can dam-

Bites

age the skin, heart, and circulation. These bites can also affect the clotting system and blood pressure. Certain venoms can paralyze victims, impair their ability to breathe, or cause internal hemorrhaging.

Coral snakes produce venom that overstimulates the nervous system. This can lead to seizures and impair a patient's ability to breathe.

What To Look For

- Overall weakness.
- Pain and swelling around the wound. Coral snake bites cause burning pain.
- Pallor or cold, clammy skin (indicates internal hemorrhaging).
- Swelling, blisters, or bruises around the wound.
- Numbness or "pins and needles" feeling in the mouth, fingers, and toes.
- Nausea, vomiting with subsequent chills, and fever. Coral snake bites can cause subsequent blurred vision.
- Muscle paralysis.
- Difficulty breathing, swallowing, or speaking.
- Seizures and/or muscle twitching.

What To Do

- Call 911 immediately.
- Check breathing and pulse. Be prepared to perform CPR.
- Keep the patient calm and motionless because activity or fear can speed the spread of venom through the body.
- Remove rings, jewelry, or tight clothing.
- Gently wash wound area.
- Loosely place a constricting band (an article of clothing or an elastic bandage) between the wound and the heart to prevent the venom from entering the bloodstream. Keep the band in place until the patient receives professional medical treatment.

What Not To Do

- Don't move the patient. Movement can speed the spread of venom through the body.
- Do not let the patient eat or drink.
- Don't elevate injured limbs.
- Don't cut into the wound and try to suck out the venom. Cuts could injure tendons, nerves, and blood vessels.

Typical Treatment

Hospital treatment centers around stabilizing neurological problems, cleansing wounds, administering antibiotics, and, in severe cases, giving the patient antivenom to neutralize poisonous toxins. Antivenom must be given intravenously within a few hours of the bite and can only be administered in a facility equipped to provide intensive care.

Follow-up Care

Snake bites may produce delayed reactions. Therefore, a victim must be observed for at least eight to twelve hours after all acute problems have apparently resolved.

A victim of a coral snake bite must be hospitalized and monitored for at least two days. A physician must reexamine the wound within twenty-four hours of discharge.

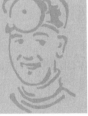

Dr. Fischer Says

It may be worthwhile to identify the type of snake involved because a patient's reaction and the treatment received may vary according to the type of snake that attacked. However, remember that time is of the essence—so don't let the identification of the snake interfere with or slow down a patient's treatment.

Spider, Scorpion, and Insect Bites

What They Are

All spiders have toxic venom, but most spider bites don't cause serious injuries. Black widow and recluse spider bites are exceptions. Black widow spider bites can cause severe muscle cramping within two hours of the bite. Brown recluse spider bites may result in severe tissue damage, ulceration, and gangrene at the site of the injury. Both black widow and recluse spider bites require quick hospital treatment.

Scorpions are found primarily in Arizona and the Southwest. They only attack humans in self-defense. They don't bite, but some inject venom by stinging with their tails. Scorpion bites may cause seizures, restlessness, agitation, rapid breathing, and drooling, which cannot be treated in the field.

Stinging insects, such as bees, wasps, hornets, yellow jackets, and fire ants can cause major emergencies even though they inject small amounts of venom. A patient who is genetically predisposed will have allergic reactions each time he/she is stung and the reaction will worsen with each ensuing sting. This is called "sensitization."

When ticks bite, they burrow into their host's body to take and infect its blood. Ticks transmit two serious diseases: Rocky Mountain spotted fever and Lyme disease. Tick bites usually don't require emergency treatment, but call a doctor to see if antibiotics are needed.

Bites by mosquitoes, horse flies, bedbugs, fleas, and lice may transmit infectious diseases of varying levels of severity. Usually, they cause only unpleasant localized reactions and patients do not become sensitized to insect bites.

What To Look For

Spider Bites

- Cramping, muscle spasms.

- Fever, chills.
- Tightness in the chest and difficulty breathing.
- Dizziness, nausea, sweating, or seizures.

Scorpion Bites
- Agitation, nausea, or vomiting.
- Muscle spasms.
- Rapid pulse and shallow breathing.
- Blurred vision or uncoordinated eye movements.

Insect Stings
- Redness, itching, and swelling around the site, the face, neck, lips, or tongue. Call 911 immediately.
- Itching, irritation, redness, flushing, or hives over the entire body (signs of severe allergic reactions). Wheezing, coughing, hoarseness, difficulty breathing or speaking may indicate swelling of the upper airway membranes, a major medical emergency.
- Plummeting blood pressure and collapse (anaphylactic shock).

Tick Bites
- Ticks clinging to or burrowing in the skin.

What To Do

Spider Bites
- Capture the spider if possible or try to determine if it's a black widow or recluse. However, don't take time away from attending to the patient.
- If it is a brown recluse spider, call 911 immediately because recluse bites can cause severe tissue damage, ulceration, and gangrene.
- Ice or place cold compresses on the bite.
- Move the patient's body so that the bite is lower than the heart.

Bites

Scorpion Bites
- Call 911 immediately. Scorpion bites can't be treated in the field so get professional help fast.

Insect Stings
- Call 911 immediately if the patient has difficulty breathing (or hoarseness) or was stung inside the mouth. If swelling of the respiratory passages develops, the patient's breathing could quickly be impaired.
- Call 911 immediately if the patient has redness, itching or swelling around the site, the entire body, face, neck, or tongue. The faster these signs appear, the more severe the emergency.
- Remove the stinger with a sharp blade and wash the area with soap.
- Find out if the patient is sensitized. Sensitized patients usually carry an insect sting kit with a "pen" that injects epinephrine. For less sensitive patients, place a thick paste of meat tenderizer and water (or even mud) directly on the wound to reduce pain, itching, and swelling.
- Apply ice packs to the wound to slow the absorption of venom into the tissues.
- Give less sensitive patients an antihistamine orally (For example Benadryl® 25 mg). Have a physician examine the patient ASAP because delayed allergic reactions could occur within the next twenty-four hours.

Tick Bites
- Remove the tick with tweezers, a knife, or a needle.
- Gently pull the tick's entire body off by its head.
- Wash the wound and apply antiseptic.
- Consult a physician immediately to see if antibiotics such as tetracycline would be appropriate.

What Not To Do
- Don't try to squeeze out insect stingers with your fingers.
- Don't squeeze a tick's body.

Typical Treatment
Spider Bites

In most cases, patients are given muscle relaxants such as Valium®. Antivenom will be used only in severe cases and usually provides relief in two to three hours.

Scorpion Bites

Intravenous fluids and medications may be given to prevent cardiac and neurological damage. Antivenom is not administered.

Insect Bites

A patient with swelling of the breathing passages will immediately receive intravenous epinephrine. Nasal oxygen, intravenous antihistamines, and, on occasion, intravenous steroids will be provided. The patient will undergo close observation in the intensive care unit for several days. A patient who only suffered localized skin reactions may receive the same medications (epinephrine, antihistamines, steroids) by injection or pills.

Tick Bites

Removal of the tick is the highest priority. If Rocky Mountain spotted fever or Lyme disease is common in the area, a patient may be given oral antibiotics such as tetracycline.

Follow-up Care
The key to controlling spider, scorpion, and insect bites is avoidance: either stay indoors or spray sparingly with pesticides. A sensitized patient should carry an insect sting kit whenever he/she might be exposed to any stinging insects. Sting kits con-

tain a "pen" filled with epinephrine, which can prevent life-threatening allergic reactions. Epinephrine is also effective for patients with life-threatening allergic reactions to food.

Dr. Fischer Says

On my first visit to Yosemite Valley, I witnessed an English tourist being stung by a bee. Within minutes, his face and lips blew up like a red balloon. Luckily, we were able to get him to the National Park hospital within a few minutes, where they were able to stabilize his condition.

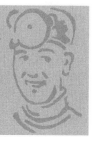

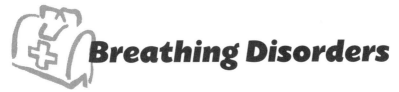

Breathing Disorders

What They Are

Shortness of breath is a symptom of a wide variety of conditions that affect the heart, lungs, circulation, and metabolism. To operate, our bodies depend on a process called respiration, which delivers an uninterrupted supply of oxygen to our cells and removes carbon dioxide. If our oxygen intake drops, our bodies try to compensate by increasing the heart and breathing rate. A patient struggling for air may develop visibly abnormal intake patterns such as using his/her shoulders, ribcage, or abdominal muscles to breathe.

Normally, we breathe eighteen times each minute in a regular, calm pattern. Anything that hinders normal circulation and delivery of oxygen can significantly increase this rate.

What To Look For

- Rapid breathing, shortness of breath.
- Breathing through pursed lips—often related to emphysema, a disorder worsened by long-term cigarette smoking.
- Speaking one syllable at a time—indicating severe respiratory distress.
- Wheezing—a sign of asthma or "water in the lungs."
- Blue lips, fingertips, or tongue (cyanosis)—a sign of poor oxygen circulation.
- Inability to breathe while lying flat—if the patient is sitting up and struggling for air, it is usually due to severe congestive heart failure (also called pulmonary edema or "water in the lungs").

Breathing Disorders

- Agitation or lethargy—signs of impaired delivery of oxygen to the brain.
- A choking noise (stridor) when the patient inhales.

What To Do

- Call 911 immediately if the lips, fingertips, or tongue turn blue and the chest wall doesn't seem to be moving. Perform CPR if needed (see p. 173).
- After you call 911, don't leave the patient alone because respiratory emergencies can worsen within seconds and you may need to perform CPR.
- Verify that the patient took prescribed medication as scheduled (for example, inhalants for asthma patients and oxygen for emphysema sufferers).
- Check the patient for signs of upper airway obstruction. Obstruction due to severe allergic reaction, certain childhood infections (such as croup), or from choking on food may be causing the shortness of breath.

What Not To Do

- Don't let the patient out of your sight.

Typical Treatment

Usually, the patient's history of respiratory problems and a physical exam will reveal the cause of his/her breathing problem. Other tests that may be ordered include arterial blood gas (to measure oxygen, carbon dioxide, and pH), chest Xrays, electrocardiograms, spirometry (to measure the patient's ability to expel air from the lungs), and hemoglobin levels (to check for anemia).

Respiratory distress can also be attributable to heart problems (heart attacks, heart rhythm disturbances, congestive heart failure, angina), asthma, high blood pressure, blood clots in the lungs, allergic reactions, choking, carbon monoxide exposures, and anxiety attacks. Rarer causes include collapsed lungs, botulism, and sickle cell disease.

Follow-up Care

Further treatment will vary in accordance with the cause and the severity of the patient's specific respiratory emergency.

Dr. Fischer Says

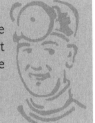

"You have no idea how frightening it is to be short of breath," one of my most brilliant professors, Dr. Sidney Tessler, a lung specialist at Maimonides Medical Center, would remind us. Therefore, take any sign of respiratory distress seriously and act quickly.

Burns

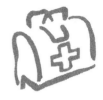

What They Are

Our skin keeps us warm, waterproof, and free from external infections. More than ninety percent of burns occur at home and are minor, but a small percentage may be life-threatening. Burn patients may suffer fluid loss, reduced body temperature, and sepsis (bacteria multiplying within the bloodstream). The extent of injury depends on the duration, location, temperature, and type (chemical or thermal) of burn.

Burns disrupt body cell functions, hormonal balance, acid-base chemistry, and blood pressure. Inflammatory chemicals, such as histamine, are released that may extend the area of injury beyond the margins of the original burn.

Superficial burns irritate exposed nerve endings and are usually painful. Deeper burns, including those caused by scalding water, kill cells and destroy arteries, veins, and nerves. As a result, a patient may not feel any pain.

Exposure to fire, smoke, and ash particles may damage the upper airways, obstruct the flow of oxygen to the lungs, and replace it with deadly carbon monoxide.

Burns are classified according to depth: full thickness, partial thickness, and first degree. Full-thickness burns go all the way to the bone; partial-thickness burns penetrate the skin, but do not reach the bone, and first-degree burns injure only the outermost layer of skin.

What To Look For

- Redness, swelling, and blistering of the affected skin.
- If a patient is coughing, wheezing, or hoarse, call 911 immediately because the upper airways may be burned or filled with carbon monoxide.

- Seepage of tissue fluid. Seepage from extensive burns can cause a drop in blood pressure and impair circulation to the heart, brain, and kidneys.

What To Do
- Separate the victim from the source of the burns.
- Call 911 immediately.
- Remove any affected articles of clothing.
- Check the patient's heart and breathing rate (See page 171). If the patient has no pulse or is not breathing, immediately begin CPR. (See page 173).
- Cover burns with cool, clean towels or sheets to return the skin's temperature to normal and protect sensitive, damaged skin.
- Remove watches, belts, rings, and jewelry that can retain heat and impair circulation to the arms and legs.
- For chemical burns, pour large amounts of tap water over the area.
- Keep injured tissue moist and cool with tap water, but don't apply ice because it could reduce body temperature too much.
- Check for damage to breathing passages, especially when a great deal of smoke, gas, steam, or fumes is present. The patient may be coughing up soot or blackened sputum indicating breathing passage damage.

What Not To Do
- Don't apply ointments or cover the burn with butter, creams, lotions, or other remedies.
- Don't cover the wound with bandages or any type of material that may stick to the fragile outer layers of skin.

Typical Treatment
If the patient is unconscious or his/her oxygen supply has been impaired, CPR may be required.

Burns

A patient burned on the mouth, tongue, nose, or face may need intensive care treatment for upper airway scalding or "water in the lungs" (pulmonary edema).

For deep or large burns, intravenous fluids will be needed to prevent circulatory collapse, brain damage, and kidney failure.

If blood tests reveal carbon monoxide poisoning, high amounts of oxygen will be given for several hours.

After the patient's blood pressure and respiratory status stabilize, dying skin may be removed surgically to prevent bacterial growth and scarring that could constrict the arms, legs, or chest. Intravenous morphine is often prescribed for massive burns.

Burn care specialists will determine what specific dressings, topical antibiotics, or surgery are appropriate. A patient will be hospitalized for several days and longer if kidney or heart damage has been incurred.

Follow-up Care

A patient with minor burns usually does not require hospitalization. However, the patient must be reexamined within twenty-four hours by a physician and specially trained nurses. A seriously injured patient will require more intensive follow-up after hospitalization. The healing process will be monitored and evaluated for three or four weeks. Scarring may be removed or improved by cosmetic surgery and skin grafting.

Dr. Fischer Says

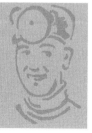

Immediately assess the patient's breathing. If he/she is coughing up charcoal-like material or is not speaking normally, call 911 and be ready to perform CPR. The patient's upper airways could be inflamed, swollen, and blocked, which could prevent breathing.

Choking

What It Is

Two separate tubes or passageways sit at the back of our mouths: the esophagus, which sends food and liquids to the stomach and intestines, and the windpipe (trachea), the airway through which air enters the lungs. These two passageways are not intended to be open at the same time so a small membrane, the epiglottis, seals the windpipe when we swallow.

When people simultaneously eat, drink, breathe, talk, and don't adequately chew their food, the epiglottis may be overwhelmed. Food meant for the digestive tract may slip into the windpipe where it gets trapped. Young children can inhale small objects into their tracheas: beans, nuts, peanuts, erasers, pieces of toys, etc.

Coughing often dislodges obstructing objects, but victims can also hyperventilate and unintentionally force foreign bodies further down the windpipe. When the upper airway isn't completely blocked, victims may still be able to breathe. However, when the windpipe is totally obstructed, air cannot pass, and victims can choke to death (the heart and brain cannot survive without oxygen for more than a few minutes). Mouth-to-mouth breathing is ineffective since foreign bodies block the entry of air into the lungs.

What To Look For

- Coughing, gasping for air, and/or clutching the throat.
- Fast and deep breathing.
- Change in the patient's voice (partial obstruction).

Choking

- Inability to talk (total obstruction).
- Wheezing (from trying to force air around the trapped object).
- Blue fingers, lips, and face.
- Collapse, unconsciousness.

What To Do
Conscious Patient
- If the patient can't talk, breathe, or cough perform the Heimlich Maneuver (abdominal thrusts).
- Call 911 immediately if he/she can talk, cough and breathe without assistance. Allow an alert patient with partial obstruction to try to clear the blockage on his/her own. Keep the patient erect, with his/her head leaning slightly forward.

Abdominal Thrusts (Heimlich Maneuver).
1. Stand directly behind the patient.
2. Wrap your arms around the patient's waist.
3. Clasp your hands above the navel under the ribcage so your thumb is pressing against the patient's abdomen. Be sure your hands are several inches below the lower tip of the patient's breastbone.
4. Pull inwards and upwards five (5) times in succession.
5. After each cycle of five (5) thrusts, gently sweep the patient's mouth with your finger to see if the object has popped out and can be removed.
6. Repeat the cycle of five (5) abdominal thrusts until the object dislodges, the person becomes unconscious or collapses, or emergency personnel arrive.

Unconscious Patient
- Call 911 immediately.
- If a patient inhaled vomit, turn the victim on his/her stomach with the head as far

down as possible. This should move the tongue forward and allow gastric contents to empty out of the mouth, not into the lungs. Then proceed as follows:

1. Turn the patient on his/her back and kneel alongside his/her hips facing the patient's head.
2. Deliver five (5) abdominal thrusts (Heimlich Maneuver) by:

   A. Pressing the heels of your hands above the patient's navel, several inches under the ribcage. Be sure your hands are below the lower tip of the breastbone.
   B. Pushing inwards and toward the shoulders five (5) times in succession.
   C. After each cycle, gently sweep the patient's mouth with your finger to see if the object has popped out and can be removed.
   D. Repeating the cycle of five (5) abdominal thrusts and checking the patient's mouth until the obstructing object is dislodged, the person becomes conscious, or emergency personnel arrive.

Choking Infants
- Place the child on his/her back.
- Place two (2) fingers between the navel and rib cage and push downwards and towards the shoulders several times.
- Check the child's mouth to see if the object popped out and can be removed. Proceed cautiously because it's easy to push objects back into the trachea. Continue until help arrives.

If You Are Choking
- Stand facing the back of a chair or over a railing.
- Place your fist between your navel and rib cage.
- Lean downward quickly into the chair or railing so that your fist presses into the abdomen and upward toward the shoulders.

- Repeat until you feel the object pop out, until you can breathe normally, or until help arrives.

What Not To Do

- Don't do anything other than call 911 if a patient is talking, coughing, and breathing normally.
- Don't try to remove partial obstructions. You could force an unstable blockage further down and create a total obstruction.
- Don't administer blows to the patient's back because they could push the object further down the windpipe.

Typical Treatment

Ambulance personnel will try to dislodge the foreign body and will give the patient intravenous fluids and oxygen.

A tracheotomy (puncturing of the front of the throat to allow air to enter the lungs) may be required if an object is still lodged in the upper airway.

A seriously impaired patient will be hospitalized for a day or two to insure that he/she hasn't suffered lung damage or pneumonia. After Xrays are taken, a pulmonologist (lung doctor) may inspect the upper airways and lungs with a specialized fiberoptic camera.

Follow-up Care

After an obstruction has been removed, the patient should sit quietly for a few minutes. Further care isn't usually required because momentary choking seldom causes significant cardiovascular or neurological damage. The patient should see a doctor immediately after a choking episode. Rib fractures and liver damage are rare, but possible, side effects of using the Heimlich Maneuver.

Dr. Fischer Says

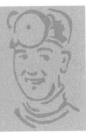

Choking most frequently occurs at restaurants or social occasions when people eat, drink, and get too merry. If you forget what to do, most restaurants have instructions posted that you can follow. Your local Red Cross holds periodic classes on how to assist choking patients; you are strongly urged to attend!

Cold Exposure
(Hypothermia)

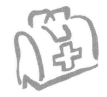

What It Is

When our body is cold, we reflexively shiver to increase our blood flow, which delivers heat to our muscles. When our body temperature falls below 95 degrees, hypothermia occurs. In response, our respiratory, heart, and brain functions slow dramatically in order to keep us alive. In effect, our vital organs go into hibernation, so hypothermia victims can survive for hours under frigid conditions.

Hypothermia is usually caused by exposure to freezing weather. It can also result from lengthy surgery (patients lose warm fluids in cold operating rooms), malnutrition, severe burns, and dehydration. Loss of tissue fluid or blood, which normally spread heat through the body, can dangerously lower body temperature. Blood-borne infections, major trauma that entails excessive bleeding, and conditions that cause extremely low blood pressure also impair the delivery of heat to our tissues.

What To Look For

- Blue lips.
- Shivering.
- Unresponsiveness, confusion, or disorientation.

What To Do

- Call 911 at once, *even if the patient seems dead*, has blue lips, isn't breathing, or has no pulse. (Hypothermia victims can only be revived if they are transported immediately to an intensive care facility.)
- After notifying 911, begin CPR (see p. 173).

- For an awake and responsive patient, check breathing and pulse every few minutes.
- Before the ambulance arrives, move the victim from the cold area, if possible.
- Replace wet clothing with dry, warm blankets, sheets, or similar coverings.

What Not To Do

- Don't feed the patient because hypothermia usually shuts off stomach, intestinal, and kidney functions. The patient could become nauseous and, if lying on his/her back, could choke on vomit.

Typical Treatment

Hypothermia, even when severe, is often reversible. The patient will be warmed with specialized blankets, heat lamps, heated oxygen, and warm intravenous and gastrointestinal fluids. As the body temperature rises, the patient will be monitored for infection, kidney and liver failure, muscle destruction, heart rhythm disturbances, and blood chemistry disorders.

It may take several days after the patient begins circulating the usual quota of warm blood for the kidney, liver, and general metabolic functions to return to normal. In extreme cases, hemodialysis may be required. Hemodialysis involves placing catheters in the patient's abdomen to remove accumulated metabolic waste and restore the acid/base balance.

Recovery usually takes several days but may last several weeks for a patient with multi-system involvement and complications.

Follow-up Care

The patient should be reexamined by his/her personal physician within a few days of discharge from the hospital. Thereafter, recovery should be monitored with periodic blood tests and EKGs. A patient who was in critical condition usually requires several weeks of outpatient evaluation.

Dr. Fischer Says

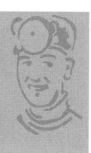

Usually, we picture stranded mountain climbers, skiers, or boating-accident patients as the typical hypothermia victims. However, hypothermia more commonly strikes the intoxicated or mentally ill who are found shivering or comatose on freezing streets. Often, these patients have wet or inadequate clothing. Alcohol, drugs, or medication may have depleted their body heat or slowed their metabolism.

Cuts and Bruises

What They Are

The skin is the body's main protective surface. Cuts (lacerations) and scrapes (abrasions) provide openings through which infections can enter the body and precious bodily fluids can seep out. These injuries primarily involve the hands, face, and scalp.

Bruises are superficial injuries of the blood vessels in the outermost skin layers. They do not provide an entry to deeper tissues and do not require antibiotics or suturing. Bruises that form small collections of blood under the skin (hematomas) usually disappear in a week or two.

Approximately twelve million wounds are treated every year in the U.S.A., accounting for ten percent of all emergency room visits. When we are cut or bruised during major traumas, such as fractures or head injuries, the potentially more serious injuries are examined and treated first.

Patients with diabetes, poor circulation, or suppressed immune systems (for example, those taking steroids) are more prone to skin infections. Infections are also more likely in injuries to the hands and feet.

Contaminated minor skin breaks can result in abscesses or cellulitis—dangerous bacterial growth in the deeper tissue layers.

Cuts and bruises may be signs of other medical conditions: sudden collapse due to heart problems, alcoholism, blackouts, epilepsy, and even child abuse. These conditions may require greater attention than the cuts or bruises themselves.

What To Look For

• Breaks in the skin.

Cuts and Bruises

- Bleeding.
- Bacterial contamination. Find out what caused the injury because dirty objects—most commonly soiled ones—can cause infection.
- Foreign objects in the wound (glass fragments, thorns, or splinters).
- How much time passed since the injury. Wounds should be examined as quickly as possible (within six hours) to prevent infection and promote healing.
- Infection: redness (including red streaks leading away from wounds), swelling, skin warmth, fever, pus, and pain.

What To Do

- For cuts with little or slight bleeding, immediately place a sterile gauze pad or large bandage over the wound to stop the bleeding and prevent bacterial contamination.
- Remove all clothing, rings, and jewelry from the affected area.
- When blood is flowing from a wound, gently place direct pressure over the wound. Elevate cut arms or hands as high as possible when transporting the patient to the hospital. Act promptly. Open wounds can become seriously infected within six to twelve hours, and sealing or bandaging them may inadvertently cause rapid bacteria growth. Surgery can't be performed on infected areas; these must be initially treated with antibiotics and surgery delayed until the healing process has started.
- Puncture wounds rarely need surgical closure, but can easily become infected.

What Not To Do

- Don't apply hydrogen peroxide, iodine, or any antibiotic creams or lotions to lacerations. They could enter the bloodstream and delay healing by injuring or over-moisturizing the area.
- Don't attempt to treat infections; leave it to emergency workers.
- Don't apply tourniquets because they can compress the blood supply to the injured area.

Cuts and Bruises

Typical Treatment

After protective coverings are removed, the extent of the injury will be determined. Minor, uninfected lacerations inflicted in the past few hours will be cleansed and sutured, stapled, or taped. Before treatment, a local anesthetic may be injected to numb the injured area. If nerves, tendons, bones, or blood vessels were injured, more extensive surgical treatment will be required.

Lacerations more than twelve hours old usually won't be sutured because they are presumed to be infected. Xrays may be needed if foreign bodies such as glass, metal, or gravel entered the lacerated area. Instead of suturing, the wound will be examined and cleansed with sterile water. Dead skin—fragments that have lost their blood supply—will be removed and wounds will be allowed to heal without surgery. Patients will be required to take antibiotics for at least a week. This is called secondary closure. A patient who hasn't received tetanus toxoid vaccinations in five to ten years will get booster shots. Wounds will be dressed with petrolatum ointment, gauze and bandages. Several follow-up appointments will be scheduled for wound inspection and care.

Follow-up Care

Wound areas may be gently cleaned twenty-four hours after being sutured, but bathing and soaking should be avoided. Lacerations should be checked within thirty-six hours for possible infection and to monitor the healing process. At that time, the wound should be redressed.

Sutures should be checked in four days and, if no complications exist, they will be removed in seven to ten days. Sutured wounds that are healing should be inspected frequently during the next two to three weeks until they are completely mended. Most lacerations heal within three to four weeks.

Dr. Fischer Says

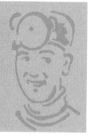

Get cuts and bruises examined quickly. When injuries are treated in the first six hours, the risk of infections decrease and the odds for successful healing increase. The signs of infections usually appear in the first four days, so be on guard. If the wound aches, burns, becomes inflamed, or develops pus, get prompt treatment.

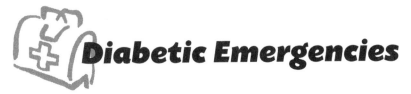

Diabetic Emergencies

What They Are

Diabetes is classified in two categories:

Type 1 diabetes, which is rare but severe, is the permanent absence of insulin (the hormone that sends sugar into cells and gives us energy). Instead of entering muscle and liver cells, sugar is released into the bloodstream. The onset of type 1 diabetes is almost always sudden and dramatic. A Patient who was fine is suddenly in an intensive care unit fighting for his/her life.

Type 2 diabetes, accounts for ninety-five percent of all cases. It occurs when the pancreas does not put out sufficient insulin or the insulin it produces is ineffective ("insulin resistance"). This is usually due to obesity, inactivity, and a genetic predisposition to the illness itself. A patient may not develop symptoms until the disease has caused major damage.

If uncontrolled, both forms of diabetes cause a dangerous rise of sugar in the bloodstream. Normal blood glucose ranges from 80 to 110 milligrams per 100 ccs. of blood (except when we eat). Emergencies usually occur when it dips below 60 mgs. (if too much medication is taken) or if it soars above 400.

Infection, stress, pregnancy, severe burns, trauma, and overeating can also elevate a diabetic's glucose. A patient can get "insulin reactions" if he/she doesn't eat enough after taking prescribed diabetic medications. Excessive sugar enters the muscles, leaving too little for the brain to function effectively.

Cardiovascular diseases, such as heart attacks, angina pectoris, and strokes are

Diabetic Emergencies

more prevalent among diabetics. Diabetes may also incur organ-specific emergencies including retinal detachment, kidney failure, and leg ulcerations.

What To Look For
- Excessive drinking of water, urination, and fatigue.
- Check for a diabetic emergency bracelet, which most diabetics wear.
- The inability to walk or move (may indicate low glucose in patients who have taken too much medication).
- Severe dehydration in frail, elderly diabetics (may indicate very high glucose).
- Confusion, dizziness, or weakness may indicate either high or low glucose ("insulin reaction").
- Breath having a fruity scent, like apricot jam. Immediately call 911 because it may indicate diabetic ketoacidosis, an emergency where the lack of insulin is so severe, and glucose so high, that fat molecules are released into the blood to supply energy to the cells.
- Rapid breathing, nausea, vomiting, and abdominal pain (diabetic ketoacidosis).

What To Do
- If the patient appears nearly comatose (due to an "insulin reaction" or overmedication) or seems to be slipping into a coma, give fruit juice, soda, or milk as soon as possible. If glucose is not restored within minutes, brain cells can die.
- If the patient drinks water and urinates excessively, call 911 or the doctor because his/her glucose may be elevated and dehydration or ketoacidosis could develop.

What Not To Do
- Don't confuse a diabetic emergency with intoxication. Always check to see if the patient has a diabetic bracelet.
- Don't minimize a diabetic's chest pain. A diabetic may develop serious heart problems with minimal or no symptoms.

Typical Treatment

Paramedics usually administer concentrated glucose intravenously for severely low sugar due to overmedication. An unresponsive, nearly comatose patient will improve within minutes and further treatment may not be needed.

A patient with extremely high glucose (over 400) will be hospitalized and given intravenous fluids and insulin injections to treat dehydration, lower sugar, and correct blood chemistry imbalances. A patient with ketoacidosis will be monitored in the intensive care unit for several days and hourly blood tests may be required.

A Type 2 diabetic with less severe complications will be hospitalized for several days to adjust his/her medication regimen and diet.

Follow-up Care

The patient should see his/her physician for blood testing a week or two after being discharged from the hospital. Blood tests may identify problems with the patient's diet, medication regimen, and other contributing factors such as infections.

Dr. Fischer Says

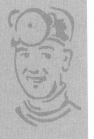

In Latin diabetes mellitus means " sweet flow of water" because physicians in ancient Rome diagnosed diabetic emergencies by tasting patients' urine. Sweet-tasting urine indicated a metabolic crisis. Diabetes has grown to epidemic proportions in the U.S., and millions more are expected to develop it in the next few years. Diabetics know how to check their sugar levels. Do you? If a diabetic is near and dear to you, learn to check sugar levels. You could save a life.

Diarrhea

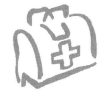

What It Is

Patients with diarrhea have watery, loose, unformed stools or a dramatic increase in the number of their daily bowel movements. Severe diarrhea can become a medical emergency if it causes dehydration, low blood pressure, and electrolyte imbalances (particularly of potassium) that can damage vital organs.

Diarrhea can be brought on by a wide variety of infectious agents including viruses (particularly in infants), bacteria (salmonella, shigella), and protozoa (amoebas, giardia). It can also be due to severe gastrointestinal illnesses (ulcerative colitis, Crohn's disease), stress ("irritable bowel syndrome"), or the side effect of medical treatments (radiation therapy for cancer) or medications (antibiotics, chemotherapy).

Food poisoning from eating contaminated or spoiled food (usually mayonnaise or creamy pie filling) is another common cause of diarrhea. Symptoms usually appear within eight hours of intake, but they may not begin until several days later.

What To Look For

- Watery, loose, unformed stools (especially if lasting more than three days).
- Dramatic increase in the number of bowel movements.
- Nausea.
- Vomiting.
- Fever.
- Abdominal cramping.
- Inability to stand or unsteadiness.

- Lightheadedness, faintness, or dizziness.
- Gas.
- Bloatedness or abdominal swelling.
- Abdominal pain.

What To Do
- Call 911 when patients complain of severe muscle cramps or cannot stand.
- If the patient feels faint, light-headed, dizzy, or unsteady on his/her feet, call his/her doctor at once. The doctor may call an ambulance or direct you to call one.

What Not To Do
Don't administer over-the-counter antidiarrheal medications when patients have severe diarrhea or cramps. Only physicians should direct their use. In infectious diarrhea, the body is trying to rid itself of offending bacteria and toxins. So stopping the diarrhea will keep poisonous bacteria in the body where they can multiply and overwhelm the intestines' defenses. Inappropriately administering medication could actually prolong the duration and severity of the patient's diarrhea.

Typical Treatment
Patients with minimal symptoms usually will not require treatment. However, the elderly may incur unrelated cardiovascular complications if fluid loss isn't corrected. Therefore, hospital treatment will be needed, which usually consists of giving intravenous fluids, identifying the cause of diarrhea, and administering antibiotics, potassium or antidiarrheal medications.

A patient showing no symptoms after eight to twelve hours of ER observation is usually discharged, which is the typical scenario with food poisoning. When a patient doesn't improve or has very low blood pressure, hospital admission will be necessary. The patient's blood will be tested to check the severity of the infection (for high white blood cell count) and potassium loss. Stool samples will also be analyzed for blood, which may indicate severe gastroenteritis or other serious diseases (ulcerative colitis or colon cancer). Melena, foul-smelling, black tarry stool, is usually due to a bleeding ulcer.

Follow-up Care

In most cases of infectious diarrhea follow-up is rarely needed and a patient is seldom hospitalized for more than a few days. Patients who have underlying diseases that caused their diarrhea should undergo diagnostic tests (colonoscopy or upper GI series) and specific treatment for those disorders before their condition can be controlled.

Dr. Fischer Says

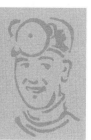

Don't treat the early stages of diarrhea with over-the-counter medications because you may actually prolong and intensify it. If diarrhea strikes while you are traveling, drink fluids to balance fluid loss and rest in bed until the crisis passes, which usually runs six to eight hours. Try to identify and avoid the offending food.

Drowning

What It Is

Inhaling water rather than air can cause unconsciousness or death from lack of oxygen (asphyxiation). When the lungs fill with water, normal chest expansion is restricted and circulating oxygen decreases. This can make the blood more acidic and cause brain damage.

Drowning is often preventable. Usually, the first rescuers are not medical personnel. Victims are often healthy children who cannot swim, but about one third of all drowning cases involves swimmers who are overwhelmed by cold or dangerous waters, intoxicated by drugs or alcohol, or suffer sudden heart attacks.

What To Look For

- Check if the patient is breathing.
- If the patient is not breathing, check for a pulse in the neck (see instructions on p. 172).

What To Do

- Remove the patient from the water ASAP! Trained personnel, such as lifeguards or paramedics, may begin treatment while the patient is still in the water.
- Place the patient on his/her back and tilt his/her head slightly back. If the patient has no pulse, begin CPR (see CPR instructions on p. 173). The need for CPR is more urgent if the patient was underwater for more than 30 seconds.
- Call 911 to assist in CPR, provide oxygen equipment, and administer necessary medication.

Drowning

- If the patient has a pulse, immediately start mouth-to-mouth (or mouth-to-nose) ventilation, one breath per three to four seconds (see directions for mouth-to-mouth ventilation on p. 174). Mouth-to-mouth breathing may stimulate the victim's respiratory center and bring immediate improvement.
- Check continually to see if the patient is reviving or breathing on his own.

What Not To Do

- Don't try to squeeze water from a patient's lungs by applying abdominal or chest pressure. The patient may have swallowed large amounts of water that could be forced from the stomach into respiratory passageways, worsening his/her condition.
- Don't attempt the Heimlich maneuver. It does not help drowning victims and will impede CPR.

Typical Treatment

Oxygen will be provided as soon as possible and a patient in serious condition will be put on mechanical ventilation. Inhaling large quantities of water can damage lung tissue and the fluid overload can impair the patient's circulation.

Specialized blood tests (arterial blood gases) will measure how much oxygen and carbon dioxide the patient is circulating as well as his/her acid base status. Imbalances will be corrected during continuous intensive care monitoring.

A patient rescued from icy or freezing cold water may require treatment for hypothermia (see Cold Exposure at p. 55).

Although chest Xrays can diagnose pneumonia or lung damage, they will not show whether the patient's oxygen circulation is adequate or if all water has been removed.

Follow-up Care

A patient with balanced arterial blood gases is usually discharged within one to two days. However, a patient who suffered lung, heart, or brain damage will require frequent follow-up.

Cardiovascular and respiratory complications (heart attack, pneumonia, or arrhythmia) may occur at any time so intensive care must continue for several days until the patient is out of danger.

Dr. Fischer Says

Practice finding the carotid artery in the neck and taking a pulse. The carotid artery is located right under the angle of the jawbone. Take the pulse by touching one side at a time.

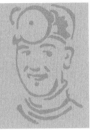

Electrical Injuries

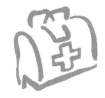

What They Are

When our skin's surface is struck by more than 600 volts of electricity, it we die. The voltage can enter the body, penetrate deeply, and kill tissue in its path. Although bones can withstand high temperatures, adjacent muscles, nerves, and blood vessels can be destroyed by strong electrical charges. Patients with deep tissue damage often exhibit minimal external signs of injury.

The skin's resistance to electricity is lowered by water and even sweating. As a result, over half the deaths from electrical injuries are caused by low voltage jolts, as in those caused when electrical appliances (radios, hair driers) fall into bathtubs.

High voltage injuries, especially those received from lightning, can cause heart damage including rhythm disturbances (usually temporary), death of cardiac muscle, and even cardiopulmonary arrest. When struck by high voltage, the body may shake with a single, powerful, muscle spasm. Renal failure can occur when fragmented muscle cells block the small tubules of the kidneys.

Direct electrical damage to internal organs is rare because the current is usually spread over the large surfaces of the chest and stomach (a "flashover"). In contrast, arm and leg injuries can be severe because less surface area absorbs the jolt. Patients can also be seriously injured when electricity ignites their clothing.

Most damage from electrical injuries occurs at the time of exposure. However, delayed complications are possible, as in subsequent blood clots that block the blood supply to a hand or foot.

Electrical Injuries

What To Look For
- Check the patient's pulse (see p. 171) and breathing rate. Start CPR if the patient is not breathing or his/her heart is not beating (see p. 173).
- Remove the patient's clothing and check for burns. The patient's internal injuries may be much worse than the visible burns you see on the surface.
- Seizures, loss of consciousness, agitation.

What To Do
- Identify, isolate, and shut off the source of electrical current.
- Call 911 immediately, even if the patient seems to have sustained only minor electrical injuries.
- Begin CPR (see p. 173) if necessary.
- Cool the affected area by gently applying towels moistened with tap water. Cover and until emergency medical personnel arrive.

What Not To Do
- Don't apply creams, antibiotics, or iodine since they could be absorbed into the bloodstream.
- Don't allow the patient to move on his/her own. There may be deep tissue damage to the muscles and/or nerves.

Typical Treatment
A patient exposed to high voltage electricity will be hospitalized and will receive continuous cardiac monitoring for several days. Those who were struck with lower voltage and experienced chest pain, pulse irregularities, amnesia, disorientation, or agitation will also be given inpatient monitoring.

Heart damage and heart rhythm disturbances are the most serious concerns. A patient with these problems may require defibrillation and intravenous medication (lidocaine, beta blockers). When the patient's cardiac condition has stabilized, the injured area is examined to make sure that muscle and nerves adjacent to bones were not damaged. Intravenous fluids will be administered if the burned tissue sustained substantial fluid loss. Physical examination and Doppler ultrasonography can determine the extent of circulatory damage.

Wounds will be cleansed with sterile fluids and burn creams that are only available by prescription. Since dead tissue is a potential source of infection, it may be surgically removed. If tissue swelling impairs circulation, fluid will be removed surgically, usually under sterile operating-room conditions. Amputation may be the only alternative if blood flow isn't restored after twenty-four to forty-eight hours of intensive effort.

The extent of injuries and recovery depends on factors such as the source of electricity, duration of exposure, amount of voltage, the anatomical path taken and the type of current involved (AC inflicts more severe damage). A patient with fluid imbalance, infection, or renal failure will require longer hospitalization.

Follow-up Care

Wounds should be reexamined every few days, preferably in a specialized burn unit. Examinations will also assess how musculoskeletal and nerve injuries are healing.

Dr. Fischer Says

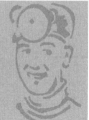

Over ten percent of deaths from burns are due to electrical injuries. Most of us have received mild jolts from touching improperly wired objects. Fortunately, our reflex to withdraw from painful stimuli prevents serious consequences.

Eye Injuries

What They Are

Most common eye injuries result from foreign objects entering and irritating the surface of the eye. Dust, sand, soil, or eyelashes usually cause minor irritation, while metal, plastic, or glass fragments can create serious damage. Even contact lenses can scratch the cornea—the clear membrane that protects the pupil and lens. Scratches can be extremely painful...and pain and irritation can often linger long after the object is removed.

As most people age, gradual changes in their eyesight occur such as nearsightedness, farsightedness, astigmatism, and aging eyes. Usually, they experience blurred vision that can be corrected by glasses. Cloudy vision can also be attributable to cataracts (whitening of the lens at the front of the eye) and glaucoma (increasing pressure inside the eyeball that produces halos around lights).

Sudden loss of vision is usually caused by diseases of the retina (the thin layer of receptor cells at the back of the eyeball), diseases of the uveal tract (the organs that bathe and defend the inner eye), or impaired circulation and oxygenation of visual pathway nerves. When retinal receptors lose their blood supply, they quickly die and cannot be replaced. Since eyesight depends heavily on normal blood circulation, illnesses that constrict or block arteries can cause sudden loss of vision. Strokes involving the retina, optic nerve, or the brain's visual processing center can also cause irreversible damage. Risk factors for such strokes include hypertension, diabetes, high cholesterol, and atrial fibrillation, which can cause dangerous blood clots.

When patients see "flashing lights" or suddenly lose vision as if a curtain was raised before them, they usually have retinal detachment (the retina peeling off the back of the eye). Retinal detachment is often caused by uncontrolled diabetes and is a major cause of blindness.

Less threatening eye emergencies include conjunctivitis (generalized redness of one or both eyes), sub-conjunctival hemorrhages (small, benign collections of blood that do not cover the pupil), and styes (infections of the oil gland at the root of an eyelash).

Blows to the face may break bones that support the eyeball and cause it to droop. Patients who cannot look upwards may have "blow-out" fractures and must be immediately examined, Xrayed, and CAT scanned or their eye movements could be permanently damaged.

Bell's palsy, a drooping or paralysis of one side of the face, is caused by viral infections that affect the nerve that controls some eye movements. Patients may be unable to blink one set of their eyelids. Bell's palsy is not a stroke and usually resolves on its own after about six weeks. However, Bell's palsy patients should be examined by a neurologist as a precaution.

Temporal arteritis produces a sudden loss of vision in one eye accompanied by a throbbing headache on the same side. If immediate treatment is not provided, it will result in blindness.

What To Look For
- Pain, tearing, or redness in the eye.
- Cloudy vision and headaches (glaucoma).
- Sudden loss of vision.
- Limited eye movements.
- Eyelids stuck together (bacterial conjunctivitis).
- Blood on the surface of the eyeball.

What To Do

- For irritation caused by foreign objects or toxic chemicals, immediately and slowly rinse with tap water at room temperature. Rinse from the side to avoid pouring water on the pupil itself, then call 911.
- Call 911 if the patient suffers a sudden loss of vision. Specialized eye centers are better equipped to handle ophthalmic emergencies caused by chemical or physical trauma, infections, or dislodged contact lenses.

What Not To Do

- Don't try to remove objects from the eye because you could scratch the cornea.
- Don't pour water directly on the pupil.

Typical Treatment

Minor problems such as foreign objects, conjunctivitis, and chemical exposure can be treated in most emergency rooms. The ER staff will examine the retina and optic nerve for hemorrhages, retinal detachment, and optic neuritis (a possible sign of multiple sclerosis). The front of the cornea will be stained with dye so examinations with specialized lenses can detect abrasions.

A patient with a retinal emergency, an acute form of glaucoma, or an internal hemorrhage due to diabetes should receive immediate, specialized testing, which isn't available at many small hospitals. These patients should be rushed to designated eye-care facilities where accurate diagnosis, administration of eye drops, intravenous medication (mannitol or Diamox® for glaucoma), or surgery may be needed to prevent permanent vision loss. When a stroke is suspected, a patient's vital signs will be checked and stabilized, and EKG, echocardiograms, carotid sonograms, CT scans, or an MRI may be ordered.

Antibiotic eye drops are prescribed for bacterial infections. Topical antibiotics are also prescribed for corneal abrasions and the eye may be temporarily patched.

Follow-up Care

Conjunctivitis and foreign object injuries usually heal within forty-eight hours and leave no permanent damage. After initial treatment, get a quick check up from the eye doctor to make sure that no complications arose and that the cornea wasn't scratched. Corneal abrasions can become infected and scar, so a patient should continue taking antibiotics and see an eye doctor regularly for several weeks to monitor the healing. The tiny broken blood vessels that cause subconjunctival hemorrhages usually take about two weeks to heal.

A patient whose vision was compromised by circulatory or cardiac problems will be given echocardiograms and/or Doppler sonograms to check the circulation in the main blood vessels of the neck and heart. If the patient has unstable atrial fibrillation or critically narrowed neck arteries, the blood should be thinned with aspirin, Coumadin®, or other anticoagulant.

Dr. Fischer Says

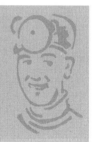

Vision occurs when patterns of light, color, shape, and movement are projected through the pupil onto the retina. From there, neurochemical impulses are transmitted through the optic nerve, where they ultimately reach the visual processing center in the brain. In emergency rooms, the phrase "curtain up" is bad news because it means retinal detachment.

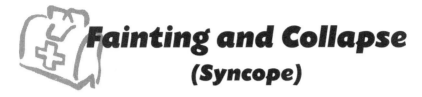

Fainting and Collapse
(Syncope)

What Are They

Fainting occurs when we suddenly and briefly lose consciousness. The oxygen supply to our brain is temporarily impaired; we then lose muscle control of our legs and collapse. Collapse is a protective mechanism because the blood flow to the head is more easily restored when patients are lying as opposed to standing.

Heart problems such as a slowed pulse (which may require a pacemaker), rhythm disturbances (such as atrial fibrillation), and structural abnormalities (defective or rigid valves) that reduce the normal blood flow can cause a sudden collapse. Fainting and collapse can be caused by severe bacterial infections, anemia, diarrhea, dehydration, and heat exposure. Either can also be the side effect of various antihypertensive and cardiac medications (diuretics, beta blockers). None of these conditions can be diagnosed or treated at home.

Fainting can be caused by episodes of intense emotion such as fear or stress. During these episodes, the heart will race and then abruptly slow, dropping blood pressure and causing the patient to collapse.

What To Look For
- Paleness.
- Cool and clammy skin.
- Complaints of dizziness or light-headedness.
- Dimmed vision.

- Unsteady gait.
- Falling or collapsing.

What To Do

All patients

- Immediately place the patient flat on his/her back with knees pointing toward the ceiling and the soles of the feet flat on the ground. Place a cool, wet cloth on the patient's forehead. See if he/she is conscious (ask "are you O.K.?") and check for a pulse.
- If the patient is unconscious, has no pulse, or doesn't respond to your question, first call 911 and then immediately begin CPR (see p. 173). Check for a pulse by feeling the inside of the wrist at the point closest to the thumb with fingers other than your thumb. Ideally, the patient will have a steady pulse of about one heart beat per second (see p. 171).
- If the patient is conscious, has a strong pulse, and says he/she feels better, keep the patient lying down for at least ten minutes, even if they want to rise.

Elderly patients

Call 911 immediately because the patient's collapse may be due to heart disease or the side effects of medication. See if the patient is conscious, check for a pulse and ask if he/she is O.K. If the patient is unconscious, has no pulse, or doesn't respond to your question, first call 911 and then immediately begin CPR. Stay with the patient until emergency personnel arrive.

Young patients

Some patients commonly have episodes called vasovagal syncope, especially during emotional or frightening experiences. These look like serious cardiovascular emergencies, but only last for a few minutes and then improve. In such instances, place the patient on his/her back with the legs or knees elevated slightly. Check for a pulse in the wrist. At first, you will probably feel a slow pulse (40 to 50 beats per minute) while the patient comes to. If the patient is conscious, has a strong, steady pulse and says that he/she is feeling better, keep the patient lying flat for at least ten minutes, even if he/she insists on getting up.

What Not To Do
Don't check the pulse or blood pressure until the patient is lying down in the position described above. Otherwise, he/she might collapse while you are checking his/her vital signs and incur additional injuries.

Typical Treatment
The ER staff will usually try to determine the cause of the collapse from the history of the event, a physical examination, lab tests (for anemia, dehydration), and an EKG (to detect heart block or other rhythm disturbances). If the collapse was due to stress or anxiety, treatment is usually unnecessary except for addressing any injuries caused by the fall.

The patient is usually monitored in ER for several hours and is not released unless the vital signs have stabilized. Longer observation, or even hospitalization, may be ordered for a patient with heart or circulatory ailments.

Follow-up Care
Usually, no further treatment or testing is necessary, unless cardiovascular disease is suspected. If heart problems are responsible for the episode, a consulting cardiologist will decide which tests to order. The options available include an echocardiogram, a stress test, or a twenty-four hour Holter monitor.

Dr. Fischer Says

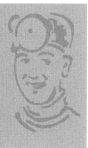

Patients who faint often say "I want to get better on my own." However, it is best to treat them as though they are seriously ill rather than minimizing the symptoms. Anxiety is a common cause of fainting. Physicians and nurses frequently encounter patients who start to pass out the moment they see a hypodermic needle coming at them. In fact, some people even get woozy when they see injections in movies.

Fractures

What They Are

Simply put, fractures are breaks in bones. Open (compound) fractures are breaks in which bone is exposed through the skin. This creates an opening for contamination and infection.

Fractures are also classified by the part of the bone injured (e.g. mid-shaft fractures), by the shape of the break (spiral fractures), and how the disrupted segments relate to each other (displaced or nondisplaced fractures). They are often accompanied by sprains (damage to ligaments that connect one bone to another), strains (injuries to tendons, the fibers that attach muscles to bones), or bruises (pockets of blood in connective tissues).

Automobile accidents can cause fractures to any of the seven vertebrae of the neck (cervical spine). They occur when cars suddenly decelerate and the passenger's neck continues its forward movement. If bone fragments injure nerves in the spinal cord, accident victims may be permanently paralyzed.

Patients who extend their arms to break falls often sustain arm and wrist fractures, ligament tears, and dislocations. Dislocations occur when the bones in a joint (the pivot point of two adjoining bones) are forced out of the joint, causing immobility and pain.

The elderly are prone to fractures of the hip joint because of their unsteadiness and fragile bones.

Children incur two unique types of injuries: greenstick fractures (incomplete breaks that rarely need surgery); and damage to the growth plate at the ends of developing long bones.

What To Look For

- Abnormally shaped arm or leg bones.
- Protruding bones.
- Extreme pain.
- Bruises.
- Swelling.
- Brown urine, a sign of massive muscle injury.

What To Do

- Call 911 immediately. Emergency personnel will stabilize the injured area and then transport the patient for additional care. They will also check for damage to patient's nerves, arteries, or veins and, in the case of rib fractures, to the lungs and heart, which may require more immediate attention than the fractures themselves.
- Check that the patient has an open airway, stable breathing, and a pulse, even when their injuries don't seem to involve critical organs. Unseen internal chest and abdominal trauma (bleeding around the lungs, ruptured spleen) may accompany serious orthopedic injuries.
- Cover exposed bone fragments with clean gauze to minimize exposure to bacterial contamination.
- Elevate and apply cold compresses to the injured area.

What Not To Do

- Don't move or touch a patient with neck injuries! Wait for the ambulance! The smallest movements can cause spinal cord damage. Emergency personnel will transport neck injury patients on specialized boards or in a brace that will immobilize their necks.

- Don't let a patient with a hip injury walk. A patient with a nondisplaced hip fracture may be able to bear weight, but doing so could cause displacement and further injury.
- Don't move fractured bones or allow others to move them. The sharp edges of fractured bones could pierce adjacent tissue, injuring nerves and blood vessels and/or piercing the skin. Instead, move both ends of the fractured bone simultaneously as a unit and place them in a straight line. If possible, support both halves by splints (see How to Make Splints, p. 182). Emergency medical personnel should perform this task unless, of course, no ambulance service is available.

Typical Treatment

Emergency personnel will first check and stabilize the patient's vital signs. Then they will try to make the patient more comfortable, and, when possible, place the fractured bone segments in alignment (reducing the fracture). They will try to align the bone as close to its original position as possible because bone tissue is continuously active and will "recognize" and unite with a separated piece. Alignment facilitates healing and in healing, the bone will hopefully replicate its original structure.

In the ER, Xrays will be taken to ascertain the extent of injury and determine whether surgery is needed. All orthopedic injuries will be compared to the unaffected side of the body. However, children frequently have both affected and unaffected limbs Xrayed so that a normal, growing bone is not mistaken for a fracture.

Broken limbs are immobilized with plaster or fiberglass casts (closed reduction). Special splints are used for fractures of the shoulder, collarbone, arm, hand, knee, and ankle.

Bleeding deep inside the hand, arm, or leg may inhibit normal circulation. When tissues cannot stretch to accommodate the increased fluid, muscles and nerves may be compressed (a compartment syndrome). Patients will feel numbness of the skin directly over the injured area and the injured limb will be pale, painful, and/or immobile. Immediate surgery is often required to relieve the compression and save the affected cells.

Shoulder dislocations are usually corrected by manually moving displaced bone back into the joint. But other dislocations, such as those to a hip, may require surgical repair. Breaks of the collarbone, nose, ribs, pelvis, and shoulder blades are usually allowed to heal on their own. Simple, nondisplaced fractures that are stabilized in casts are Xrayed over the next few weeks to monitor healing. Strains, sprains, and bruises that accompany fractures are also treated in the ER, usually with cold compresses and elevation to minimize tissue swelling.

Severe injury to an arm, leg, or hip may require surgery (open reduction) within twenty-four hours. If the injury involves an open fracture, immediate surgery (and intravenous antibiotics) will be needed. Cervical-spine fractures, especially when unstable, require prompt evaluation with CT scanning, MRIs, and neurosurgery.

A healed fracture site may become stronger than the original bone because the healing process often lays down extra new bone.

Common orthopedic emergencies include:

1. Fracture of the fifth metacarpal bone of the hand ("boxer's fracture").
2. Collarbone fracture (the most common fracture of childhood).
3. Colles' fracture (of the forearm at the wrist).
4. Pelvic fracture (often resulting in internal hemorrhage).
5. Anterior dislocation of the shoulder (treated with manipulation).
6. Rotator cuff injury (inflammation or rupture of shoulder muscles, restricting arm raising or overhead movements).
7. Hip fracture (producing shortening and outward rotation of the leg).
8. Sprain of outer ankle ligaments (the most common ankle injury).

9.   Dislocation of elbow (also due to falls, it may injure nerves and blood vessels if not quickly identified and treated).

Follow-up Care

Most orthopedic injuries do not require hospitalization, but an orthopedist (a bone specialist) should see the patient every few days until the swelling and pain begin to disappear. Orthopedists periodically reexamine and may Xray and recast patients. Patients who have not had surgery generally have good recoveries.

Patients who cannot walk without assistance will need wheelchairs, canes, or crutches. At home, the injured limb must initially be elevated above heart level. For example, if a patient's leg is broken, he/she should lie down with the leg raised so accumulated tissue fluid and blood can flow "downhill."

After surgery, patients with major vertebral or spinal fractures will remain in the hospital several days or even weeks. When their conditions stabilize, they will be transferred to a rehabilitation facility, where they will remain for several more weeks to recuperate. Seriously infected open fractures (osteomyelitis) require intravenous antibiotics, often for a month or more.

Dr. Fischer Says

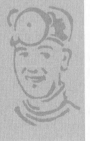

Even when Xrays are immediately taken after an injury, several types of fractures can be missed. A patient who experiences pain and discomfort within seven to ten days needs a follow-up orthopedic exam. Fractures frequently missed include those to the elbow (radial head), foot ("stress" or "march"), and wrist (navicular).

Again, don't move anyone who has neck pain after an accident, especially a high-impact injury. Don't even touch them. Wait for qualified emergency medical personnel!

Gunshot and Stab Wounds

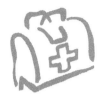

What They Are

Direct, blunt trauma and shock waves from high-velocity bullets will damage everything in their path. Bullets enter the body in a spinning, twisting motion and will break bones, rupture internal organs, and shred muscles. Tissues adjoining a wound may stretch, detach, or be torn from heat, metal, or bone fragments. A victim's outward appearance may be deceiving because internal injuries may not be apparent to untrained observers.

On the other hand, the damage from a low-velocity knife or a small caliber bullet wound is usually more apparent and localized. Victims usually incur noticeable wounds and bleeding. Perforation of a single critical organ, such as the spleen or a lung, may have rapid, fatal consequences. A severed and exposed artery anywhere in the body can create potentially deadly blood loss.

Penetrating wounds caused by knives and bullets account for almost ten percent of all ER visits in the U.S.A.

What To Look For

- A penetrating wound.
- Localized pain.
- Bleeding.
- Pale, cold, and clammy skin (from blood loss, which may be internal).
- Dizziness, unsteadiness, or collapse.
- Shortness of breath, particularly when a chest injury causes a lung to deflate.

Gunshot and Stab Wounds

Gunshot victims, especially those in their twenties or thirties, may not show any outward signs of severe internal bleeding. Whenever you find a penetrating wound to the chest below the nipples, assume that the patient has an abdominal injury.

What To Do

- Call 911 immediately. Speed is of the essence.
- Keep the victim lying down, calm, and quiet. Otherwise, a patient who is bleeding internally could faint and incur further injuries.

First aid

1. Pack the wound with clean gauze pads.
2. Apply direct pressure with a clean cloth, dressing, or gauze on a bleeding wound to stop the blood flow.
3. For arm or leg wounds, lightly wrap material, cord, or a belt around the injured appendage between the wound and the patient's head. This will reduce the blood supply to the wound area and prevent further blood loss.
4. Rinse the area with water to keep it clean. Do not scrub the area or use soaps of any kind. Infection occurs when skin bacteria are introduced into the deeper connective tissues.

What Not To Do

- Don't try to remove a bullet or knife yourself. A lodged weapon may be preventing blood loss. Removal could expose a severed artery or vein, leading to circulatory collapse.
- Don't scrub the area or use soaps of any kind.
- Don't allow the patient to stand, walk, or eat.
- Don't elevate a bleeding arm or leg because an artery may be injured and circulation of blood to the limb could be impaired.

- Don't make any assumptions about the extent of the patient's injury because a bullet's path is unpredictable. Get the patient immediate treatment.

Typical Treatment

Stabilizing the patient's vital signs is always the first priority. While doing so, the ER staff will assess the extent of the injuries. Treatment can range from cleaning and suturing the patient's wound to complex surgery, depending on the extent of the injury.

Most seriously injured patients are taken to specialized trauma centers where surgical teams are on hand. The precise treatment they provide will depend on the organs affected, the extent of the damage, and the pathway that the weapon created.

Since skin bacteria (staphylococci, for example) are pushed into the deeper connective tissues during a bullet or knife injury, patients are usually given antibiotics to take for at least one week.

Follow-up Care

Hospital staff will provide specific instructions consistent with the injuries. The wounds should be reexamined within four to seven days after the original treatment or hospital discharge, at which time most sutures can be removed. Antibiotics are usually continued for about two weeks.

Dr. Fischer Says

Consider all gunshot and stab wounds to be potentially fatal. A seemingly harmless abdominal injury might result in a ruptured spleen, leading to internal hemorrhage and shock. Young patients may lose as much as sixty percent of their blood internally without showing outward signs of injury.

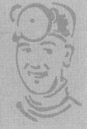

Headaches

What They Are

Although virtually everyone gets headaches, most of them are minor and over-the-counter pain remedies usually provide quick relief. However, some headaches are long lasting, resistant to pain remedies, and indicate serious medical problems that require prompt treatment.

No one knows what causes headaches, but a number of theories exist. Headaches can be attributable to the misfiring or overstimulation of pain receptors in the skull or a heightened sensitivity to normal arterial pulsations. They may also be due to high blood pressure, sinusitis, dental disease, eye (glaucoma), ear, and neck ailments, and alcohol intoxication (hangovers) to name just a few. Headaches can cause intense pain, but they usually don't produce any visible physical abnormalities. Only about four percent of all headaches result from damage to internal structures in the skull.

What To Look For

Cluster headaches

- Short bouts of pain around one eye (can waken patient from sleep).
- Intense anxiety and agitation.
- Redness in one eye (like a "shiner"), tearing, and a runny nose.

Migraine headaches

- An "aura" of flashing lights, dark spots, or jagged lines may precede the attack.
- Throbbing pain on one side of the skull that may last for hours or, in extreme cases, days.

- Sensitivity to bright lights or loud sounds.

Tension headaches
- Constricting pain, "like a knot" or like muscle spasms, over the patient's entire scalp or neck.
- Pain worsening with stress as the day progresses.

Traction headaches
- Sudden onset.
- Disorientation, unresponsiveness, or unconsciousness.
- Nausea and vomiting.
- Pain caused by abnormal collections of blood that compress brain tissue. These include intracranial bleeding (cerebral aneurysms, subdural hematoma, and subarachnoid hemorrhage), hemorrhagic strokes, and expanding mass lesions such as brain tumors.

Temporal Arteritis
- Pain on one side of forehead.
- Impaired vision or blindness affecting the eye on the same side as the pain.

Infections of the brain (encephalitis) or its covering membranes (meningitis)
- Fever.
- Nausea, vomiting.
- Stiffness of the neck.
- Confusion and delirium.

What To Do
- Call 911 immediately if the patient has neck stiffness, is vomiting, or becomes unresponsive...time is of the essence.
- Call 911 immediately if the patient is dizzy, unsteady, confused, or having the

"worst headache I've ever felt." Violent headaches that begin suddenly may indicate bleeding into the brain.

- Treat mild headaches that are not accompanied by other symptoms with over-the-counter painkillers (Tylenol®) or anti-inflammatory drugs (aspirin, Indocin, and Motrin®), bed rest in a quiet, dark environment, and cold compresses to the forehead.
- Notify the patient's doctor of newly developing headaches or changes in the usual pattern.

Typical Treatment

Often, the patient's symptoms may not accurately identify the actual headache syndrome involved. For example, a migraine can appear to be a tension headache or encephalitis may resemble a cluster headache. Therefore, the ER staff will base treatment more on patient history than on the "textbook" signs.

Patients will be questioned about the onset, location, severity, duration, and frequency of their pain; associated symptoms (nausea, vomiting, dizziness, auras, double vision, fever, or neck stiffness) and precipitating factors (medications, foods, exertion, or wine).

The most serious headaches, those associated with brain tumors or with bleeding into the central nervous system, are identified by diagnostic CT scans or MRIs. These serious conditions usually require complex neurosurgery to prevent respiratory arrest and death. On rare occasions, small holes are drilled into the skull to relieve brain swelling.

When meningitis is suspected, a lumbar puncture will be performed. The patient's spinal fluid will be examined. Antibiotic or antiviral medications will usually be started before test results come back.

Cluster headaches, unlike other headaches, often improve when patients receive extremely high concentrations of oxygen.

Headaches

When the cause of the headache is diagnosed, a variety of medications can be prescribed to address the specific type of headache. These include beta-blockers, anti-inflammatory drugs, and over-the-counter remedies. Fluid replacement and rest in a quiet, dark room are also helpful.

Patients with temporal arteritis will be given steroids.

Follow-up Care

Migraine, cluster headaches, and temporal arteritis are chronic conditions that feature relapses and pain-free intervals. In addition to over-the-counter remedies, a variety of medications are prescribed for specific headache syndromes. These include Imitrex®, ergotamine, Lithium®, beta-blockers, and anti-inflammatory drugs. Usually, a patient begins taking these drugs in the ER. Several days later, during an examination by the patient's physician, the effectiveness of the medication and its dosage will be evaluated.

If the patient is required to take medication regularly to remain pain free, his/her physician should be seen at least every four to six weeks to monitor the condition and medication.

Dr. Fischer Says

High blood pressure usually does not cause headaches. However, headaches may raise blood pressure. Severe headaches in a burn victim can indicate carbon monoxide poisoning.

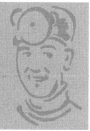

Head Injuries

What They Are

Trauma to the skull can damage or destroy brain cells and cause intracranial bleeding. Severe trauma can also cause fractures of the skull itself. Head injuries can occur during car crashes or violent attacks, but they can also follow seemingly minor injuries.

Internal swelling from head injuries can cause compression of the brain stem, the control center that regulates most of our important bodily functions. Brain stem compression can damage the respiratory center and cause death by paralyzing the diaphragm (the muscle between the abdomen and chest that enables us to breathe).

Blunt skull trauma results from blows to the head, such as those incurred during sporting events or falls. Such trauma can cause concussion, the brief loss of consciousness that may be accompanied by memory loss. Injuries associated with concussions can cause permanent brain damage, so patients who lose consciousness should receive prompt medical care.

WARNING: Seemingly mild head injuries can turn into serious problems within twenty-four hours (in rare cases, even as long as a month later). Patients over sixty-five, especially those on blood thinners, run greater risks of complications.

What To Look For

- Brief loss of consciousness.
- Inability to remember what occurred.
- Headache.

Head Injuries

- Dizziness.
- Confusion.
- Arm or leg weakness or unsteadiness.
- Speech impairment.
- Sleepiness.

What To Do

- Ask the patient's name, what day it is, and where he/she is.
- If the response is not correct, call 911 immediately.
- Patients with chronic medical conditions, especially those with hypertension and heart ailments, should be taken for prompt emergency evaluation.
- Look for blood or clear fluid in the nose or ears (often a sign of a skull fracture).
- Unequal pupil size may indicate brain stem compression.

What Not To Do

Don't give sedatives. They could complicate diagnosis and cause dangerous respiratory problems.

Typical Treatment

Emergency room personnel will document and monitor the patient's vital signs, orientation, bodily movements, ability to follow instructions, and speech pattern.

When the brain's respiratory center is injured, proper blood flow will be restored using mechanical respiration. The patient's blood pressure and pulse will be checked to determine if internal injuries such as spleen rupture or intra-abdominal bleeding were suffered. If so, intravenous fluids, medication, or surgery may be necessary.

If CAT scans detect intracranial bleeding, holes will be drilled into the skull to drain hematomas (areas of swelling due to collected blood). Draining is intended to alleviate intracranial pressure and avoid damage to the respiratory center. Cerebral compression frequently triggers a reflex that slows the pulse. If that occurs, patients will be fitted with a cardiac pacemaker.

Surgery is performed on fractured skulls only if the brain has been compressed by bone fragments (a "depressed" skull fracture).

Follow-up Care

Older patients, especially those who live alone, will usually be hospitalized and monitored for at least twenty-four hours. Young, healthy patients without concussion or amnesia are usually sent home after initial treatment, but their family and friends should monitor their conditions for at least the next twenty-four hours. If they show any of the symptoms described above, they should immediately return to the hospital.

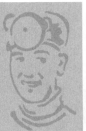

Dr. Fischer Says

Usually, impaired thinking, concentration, and memory caused by head injuries improve within a few months. Some patients may continue to have minor headaches, insomnia, and depression even though their tests reveal no abnormalities. If so, avoid medications because they could disguise potentially important symptoms.

Hearing Emergencies

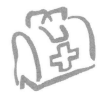

What They Are

Our ears are built to capture sound waves and funnel them to our eardrums. The captured sound waves are turned into vibrations that flow through the auditory canal to small internal bones and receptors that convert the vibrations into impulses that the brain decodes. Interruption of this process at any point can distort, muffle, or even eliminate those sounds.

The eardrum is susceptible to injury from accidents (from diving, foreign objects, and direct blows), infections, and from incorrect cleaning (inserting cotton swabs too deeply). Swimmer's ear (otitis externa) is similar to a skin infection and is usually caused by common skin bacteria (staphylococcus and pseudomonas). Infection in the central auditory canal (otitis media) occurs when upper respiratory tract infections spread through the mouth and Eustachian tube into one ear.

The inner ear controls not only our hearing, but also our balance. A connection between the inner ear and the eye muscles (through the brain) enables us to coordinate vision and balance. An infection of the inner ear is called acute labyrinthitis and is usually a complication of a cold. It produces severe vertigo (misperception of movement when an individual is motionless) and imbalance, not hearing loss.

Meniere's disease features repeated episodes of vertigo, hearing loss, ringing in the ears, and a "stuffed up" feeling. It can be a recurrent condition that lasts for decades.

The most common cause of impaired hearing occurs when thick gobs of earwax accumulate in and plug the eardrum. The wax blocks the passage of sound waves like a muted trumpet. Wax can be easily removed at your doctor's office and treatment at an acute-care facility is not necessary.

What To Look For

- *Eardrum perforations (punctures)*. Intense pain in the ear, bloody drainage, dizziness, ringing sounds, and/or hearing loss.
- *Trapped objects* in the ear such as beans, cotton swab tips, insects, and even earwax. Often, when patients try to remove objects, they push them in more deeply. To prevent infection, irritation, or perforation, have only trained medical personnel remove foreign objects.
- *Swimmer's ear* (otitis externa). Yellow drainage from the ear, pain when opening the mouth widely and often fever.
- *Middle ear infection* (otitis media). Children tugging an ear, adults experiencing hearing loss, earache, fever, and watery discharge. In severe middle ear infections, eardrums bulge outwardly (from over accumulation of inflammatory secretions) and can perforate.
- *Inner ear infection* (labyrinthitis). Complaints that "the room is spinning," nausea and vomiting, but no hearing loss.

What To Do

- Go immediately to a specialized ear/nose/throat facility, especially for perforated eardrums. *Never call 911 for ear emergencies*.
- If a specialized ear/nose/throat facility is not located nearby, go promptly to a hospital emergency room.
- If children tug at one ear or adults have hearing loss, earache, fever, and watery discharge (middle ear infection), promptly consult an ear/nose/throat specialist.

What Not To Do

- Don't remove foreign objects. You may infect, irritate, or perforate the eardrum.

Have a healthcare professional do it!
- Don't call 911 for ear emergencies.

Typical Treatment

When an eardrum is perforated but the tiny receptors in the middle ear are not damaged, further treatment usually isn't needed. Emergency personnel will rinse out the ear, prescribe antibiotic drops and schedule a follow-up exam in a few days. Ninety percent of perforations heal by themselves in three to four months, but serious perforations require immediate hospitalization, intravenous antibiotics, and surgery.

Removing foreign objects from children's ears often requires sedation. Trapped insects can be drowned by gently washing the ear with lidocaine solution or mineral oil.

Swimmer's ear is usually eliminated when topical antibiotics are applied with a medicine dropper several times a day. Normally, no follow-up is necessary.

Middle ear infections are treated with oral antibiotics (amoxicillin, Bactrim®, or erythromycin), the same drugs prescribed for bronchitis and lung infections.

Labyrinthitis responds well to meclizine, prescribed under the name Antivert®. However, since vertigo may recur (especially in Meniere's disease), it is important for a patient to quickly spot the symptoms and take meclizine to minimize the attacks.

Follow-up Care

For perforated eardrums, patients should take antibiotic drops and be reexamined in several days to monitor healing.

Middle ear infections should be checked a week after initial treatment to make sure that the structures in the auditory canal and hearing were not affected.

Dr. Fischer Says

At the Emergency Room at New York City's Cabrini Hospital, I once treated a child who was plagued by a "buzzing in one ear." Imagine my shock when I looked through the otoscope and saw a cockroach staring directly back at me. The intruder was quickly dislodged by a mineral oil bath.

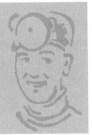

Heart Attacks

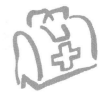

What They Are

When an artery carrying blood to the heart is blocked, the heart muscle is suddenly deprived of vital oxygen. Without oxygen, heart-muscle cells can die. When they die, the heart cannot effectively pump blood throughout the body, which crucial organs such as the brain and kidneys need to survive. Microscopic electrical misfirings can be triggered in the heart (arrhythmias). Blood and tissue fluid can accumulate in the lungs and legs (congestive heart failure).

The term "acute coronary syndrome" refers to diseases ranging from mild, chronic chest pains (angina pectoris) to deadly heart attacks (myocardial infarctions). Heart attacks claim over 500,000 deaths in the U.S.A. annually.

What To Look For

- Left-sided chest pain, central chest pain ("like an elephant standing on me"), central abdominal pain, jaw or neck pain, or left shoulder pain that may travel down the back of either or both arms.
- Heart attack pain lasts up to two hours. Pain due to chronic angina, which is provoked by exertion and relieved by rest, lasts two to twenty minutes. Exercise, cold weather, and stress can also cause chest pain.
- Possible nausea, vomiting, shortness of breath, palpitations, severe dizziness, or cold sweat on the forehead.

WARNING: *Heart attacks can occur without any of the above symptoms, especially in women*

What To Do

- Call 911 immediately. Speed is of the essence. Quick action saves most heart attack victims.
- Take the patient's pulse to determine its strength (see p. 171). If the patient has no pulse, perform CPR (see p. 173).
- If the patient has nitroglycerin, insert or spray it under the tongue.
- Give the patient a single aspirin (of at least 160 mg).

What Not To Do

Don't delay calling 911 for even a second, even if the patient has sudden cardiac arrest!

Typical Treatment

Monitored hospital confinement is needed for at least two to three days. Two tests confirm the diagnosis: the electrocardiogram, which shows the electrical damage done to heart muscle, and blood tests that identify chemicals released from dead heart cells.

Medications that will be given include intravenous nitroglycerin to open unaffected blood vessels, morphine for severe pain, beta-blockers to relax and slow the heart, and nasal oxygen to keep jeopardized cells alive.

During a heart attack, the patient's blood stream becomes thicker and stickier. Therefore, intravenous fluids and medications (heparin, streptokinase, tPA, etc.) are administered to thin blood and/or destroy large blood clots.

Strict bed rest is needed until the crisis passes.

Critically ill patients may need coronary blockages opened by high tech surgery in which clogged arteries are burrowed through (angioplasty) or replaced (coronary bypass surgery) by a blood vessel from the patient's leg or chest wall. A stent, a stainless steel tube, is inserted to open the affected artery, to keep it open, and to restore normal circulation.

Follow-up Care

Cardiac patients must begin a lifetime regimen to correct their bad habits (obesity, smoking, lack of physical exercise) and address adverse risk factors including diet, smoking, exercise, and stress management.

Patients will be put on medication including nitroglycerin, cholesterol lowering, and/or blood pressure drugs.

Most nonsurgical patients stabilize and improve within three weeks. Recovery period for surgery patients depends on the extent of the surgery.

Dr. Fischer Says

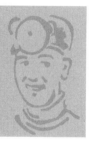

Patients who suffer heart attacks survive two-thirds of the time. It's better to err on the side of caution and assume that any severe chest symptom represents a cardiac emergency. Learn how to take a pulse and practice on your family and friends. And learn CPR as well.

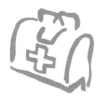

Heart Rhythm Abnormalities

What They Are

Our organs, tissues, and cells need oxygen to survive. They get oxygen from blood that circulates through the body; the supply must be regular and uninterrupted. Normally, an adult heart pumps blood in a steady, even pattern between 50 to 100 times a minute. When the heart beats less than 40 times per minute or over 150 times, the supply of blood that the heart circulates can decrease. Either abnormality can drop blood pressure significantly because the heart doesn't fill up properly.

Some patients experience "extra heartbeats," sporadic twitching of irritable heart-muscle fibers. Although they are common and usually harmless, extra heartbeats can impair circulation leading to dizziness and collapse.

When unusually large electrical disturbances spread through cardiac muscle, the heart literally stops pumping and brain cells will begin to die within three to five minutes. These disturbances can come on suddenly without warning or clue.

Abnormal or disordered electrical flow can cause ineffective pumping in the atria (the upper one-third of the heart) or the more important ventricles (the lower two-thirds of the heart). Ventricular fibrillation (muscle fiber twitching and wiggling) will usually paralyze the heart muscle and must be treated immediately. In addition, both the upper and lower heart can become electrically independent of each other, which is called heart block. More common, but less deadly, are extremely rapid impulses generated during upper-heart (atrial) fibrillation during which the heart may beat over 200 times per minute.

Heart Rhythm Abnormalities

What To Look For
- Irregular, chaotic, or extremely rapid heartbeats (palpitations).
- Shortness of breath.
- Chest pain.
- Dizziness, light-headedness.
- Dimmed vision.
- Collapse.

What To Do
- Call 911 immediately and say "This is a cardiac emergency."
- Check the patient's pulse to determine the heart rate (see p. 171). Heart rates can be influenced by the patient's age, temperature, emotions, level of fitness, and hormonal chemistries. For example, an athlete's resting pulse may be 30 to 40 beats per minute while an infant's is usually 130 to 160. Pay more attention to the symptoms listed above than to the patient's pulse rate.
- Give CPR (see p. 173) when the patient isn't breathing and the heart isn't beating. If ventricular (lower heart) tachycardia is suspected, thump the patient once sharply on the breastbone as if you were pounding on a door.

Typical Treatment
When a patient's heart has stopped, emergency personnel will try to revive him/her by giving CPR and/or applying electrical current directly to the chest wall. In less critical situations, emergency workers will try to stabilize the patient to make sure that blood flows continuously to the brain and heart. A patient being transported to the hospital will be given oxygen and possibly intravenous medication (lidocaine or atropine) to either slow, speed up, or normalize their heartbeat patterns.

At the emergency room, the patient will be given an EKG and receive continuous cardiac monitoring. The precise treatment will depend primarily on the patient's circulatory condition as well as the nature and rate of the rhythm disturbance itself.

A patient who has a very slow heart rate (usually under 50 beats per minute) will receive a pacemaker—an implanted, battery-driven, electronic device that stimulates the heart so that it beats effectively.

To control heart rhythm disturbances, intravenous medications (digitalis, beta-blockers, quinidine, Dilantin®, calcium-channel antagonists, and lidocaine) may be administered. These medications are injected slowly over several hours while the patient's response and vital signs are monitored.

Most patients with heart-rhythm disturbances will be kept for close observation at least twenty-four hours. Those with more serious or unstable conditions will remain in the intensive care unit at least a few days.

Follow-up Care

Periodic evaluation by a cardiologist is a must! Some patients will be required to continue taking stabilizing medication (propanolol, verapamil, digitalis, quinidine) for the rest of their lives. Patients with underlying coronary disease should be given stress tests, echocardiograms, or home monitoring to prevent recurrences that could prove more dangerous than the initial episode.

Dr. Fischer Says

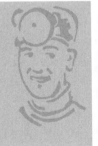

In the U.S., one quarter of all deaths from heart disorders—over 300,000 annually—are caused by electrical-flow disturbances. In evaluating a patient, assessing whether blood is circulating properly is more important than the patient's heart rhythm itself. Blood pressure collapse, which results from cardiac arrest and shock, can result from fast, slow, or chaotic heartbeats. Call 911 if this is suspected.

Heat Emergencies
(Hyperthermia)

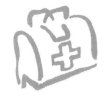

What They Are

Our cells die at temperatures of 113 to 114 degrees and never regenerate. Therefore, we have developed mechanisms that operate like thermostats to regulate our body temperature. When we get too hot, warm body fluids are sent to pores on the skin's surface where they evaporate as sweat. Conversely, we shiver when we are cold to circulate the blood that warms our tissues.

Problems arise when the body can't rid itself of excess heat. During periods of high humidity, the body retains heat because sweat does not fully evaporate. In addition, the body cannot eliminate all excessive heat caused by infection (fever), hyperactivity (epilepsy, alcohol withdrawal), certain drug use (cocaine, PCP, and amphetamines), and prolonged exposure (saunas, hot tubs, and overheated cars).

Sports enthusiasts or outdoor workers can lose too much fluid sweating in hot, humid weather and become dehydrated. Dehydration—the loss of too much body fluid and salt—decreases blood pressure and causes symptoms ranging from mild, uncomfortable heat cramps to painful muscle spasms (in the arms, legs, or upper torso), severe headache, and two potentially dangerous conditions: heatstroke and heat exhaustion.

Heatstroke occurs when the brain's thermostat is disrupted and body temperature rises above 104.9 degrees. Instead of losing heat and cooling off, heatstroke patients get paradoxically hotter, often to levels warmer than their surroundings. When body temperature is not regulated, patients' vital organ functions can be severely damaged. Older, frailer patients, infants, and the poor are especially prone to heatstroke.

Heat exhaustion is essentially severe dehydration that seldom requires hospitalization. Although it can cause damage to the heart, brain, or kidneys, patients usually recover fully.

What To Look For
- Altered mental state. Disorientation or delirium (sign of heatstroke).
- Flushed, reddened skin.
- Dry, hot skin that may be warmer than the outside temperature (sign of heatstroke).
- Total unresponsiveness (heatstroke).
- Leg muscle cramps.
- Severe headache.

What To Do
- Before calling 911, move the patient out of direct sunlight to a cool, shady spot, if possible.
- Call 911 if the patient has heatstroke. Suspect heatstroke when the patient's skin is warmer than the outside temperature (often over 105 degrees) or if the patient is delirious, disoriented, or unresponsive (comatose).
- Remove or open constricting clothing.
- Sponge cold water liberally on the skin and fan the patient.
- Gently massage the limbs to promote circulation and prevent tissue damage in the fingers and toes.
- Give water to patients with leg cramps, but insist that they drink it slowly. When emergency personnel arrive, they will administer intravenous hydration.

What Not To Do
- Don't try to cool heatstroke patients by giving them cold beverages or food; their

digestion may be impaired and they could vomit or choke.

- Don't allow an overheated patient to stand or walk on his/her own. The lower blood volume caused by dehydration may cause him/her to collapse.
- Don't give patients salt tablets because they need immediate fluid replacement.
- Don't give patients aspirin or Tylenol®, which are not helpful for heat-related emergencies.

Typical Treatment

Heatstroke is a major medical emergency that can damage many organs. For example, fluid loss and lowered blood pressure may affect tissue oxygenation and cause epileptic seizures, heart rhythm disturbances, or kidney problems. Heatstroke can impair the clotting system, damage dehydrated muscle cells, and even cause cardiopulmonary arrest.

Since heatstroke can affect many different organs, treatment will vary in accordance with each specific injury. Generally, patients will be cooled with intravenous solutions, ice packs to their armpits and groin, and possibly ice water delivered to the stomach via specialized tubing. Unless complications arise, most heatstroke patients will be kept in the intensive care unit for only a few days.

Heat exhaustion patients are usually treated with intravenous fluids and then discharged. However, cardiac patients and the elderly should be monitored for twenty-four hours after the episode, even if they are feeling better.

Follow-up Care

Heat cramps and heat exhaustion usually improve within twenty-four to forty-eight hours and rarely require further treatment.

When heatstroke is promptly treated, it generally takes at least a week to see significant improvement.

Dr. Fischer Says

Assume that a delirious, hot, bone-dry patient has heatstroke until otherwise proven. Heatstroke has a fifty percent mortality rate because of the catastrophic effects of dehydration and vital organ compromise.

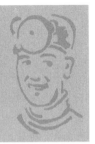

High Blood Pressure

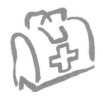

What It Is

When blood circulates through our bodies, it exerts pressure on the inside of our artery walls. In most cases, our bodies operate most efficiently when that pressure ranges between 90/60 and 120/80 (normal readings).

Sustained blood pressure of 180/110 or above can cause strokes, sudden injuries to the brain that may result in paralysis and death. High blood pressure (hypertension) can damage coronary arteries, rupture the aortic wall, and cause kidney failure, heart attacks, and pulmonary edema (water in the lungs).

Hypertensive encephalopathy, a condition that entails altered levels of consciousness and impaired vision, may occur when blood pressure readings soar to 240/140. Isolated readings that are approximately ten to twenty points above normal and that accompany severe pain, panic attacks, stimulant abuse, and testing by medical personnel ("white coat" syndrome), are called transient hypertension.

Although medical science has not been able to identify a definitive cause of high blood pressure, experts believe that the condition may be influenced by dietary indiscretion such as eating too much salt or drinking too much red wine.

Hypertension can be a silent killer that strikes the unaware. Over half of all Americans with high blood pressure don't know that they suffer from the disorder.

What To Look For

- Headache, double vision, or dizziness.
- Paralysis preventing patients from moving, talking, or even breathing (signaling a stroke, the most feared complication).

- Chest pains and palpitations.
- Nausea, vomiting.
- Confusion, disorientation, agitation, or sleeplessness.

What To Do

- Call 911 immediately if the patient has double vision, a severe frontal headache, shortness of breath, or chest pressure. Also call 911 when the elderly or diabetics exhibit these symptoms, even if their blood pressure seems normal. Delay can be disastrous.
- Call the patient's physician.
- A patient suspected of having suffered a heart attack or stroke requires urgent attention regardless of the blood pressure readings.

What Not To Do

Don't give the patient any medication until you clear it with his/her doctor.

Typical Treatment

Emergency treatment focuses on preventing or minimizing damage to the heart, brain, and kidneys. Intravenous antihypertensive medications may be administered such as nitroprusside, labetolol, esmolol, or nitroglycerin. For less urgent conditions, oral medications may be given including nifedipine, clonidine, and nitroglycerin. Treatment is usually a slow and closely monitored process because lowering blood pressure too quickly can decrease the blood flow to the heart or brain and cause permanent damage.

When hypertensive encephalopathy is promptly treated with intravenous nitroprusside, brain damage can be avoided.

A patient with a high blood pressure emergency is often admitted to a hospital "for observation." The person remains hospitalized until his/her blood pressure stabilizes at a safe level (under 140/90) and until tests verify that no cardiovascular, brain, or kidney damage has occurred.

Follow-up Care

The patient is generally put on daily medication. Blood pressure must be monitored at least twice per day and patients, and their caregivers, should learn how to take blood pressure readings.

Dr. Fischer Says

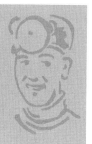

Hypertension is a huge and growing problem that affects twenty-five percent of the U.S. population and over half of our senior citizens. Unfortunately, the condition of only about twenty-eight percent of these people is treated effectively. Have your blood pressure checked regularly and, if it is high, get a home monitor and learn to take accurate readings.

Kidney Stones

What They Are

Kidney stones are pebble-sized pieces of calcium that crystallize in the small tubes of the urinary tract. They often have jagged surfaces or sharp burrs. When these stones can't flow freely "downstream" from the kidney via the ureter (the duct that conveys urine) to the bladder, blockage occurs and causes excruciating pain called renal colic. Kidney stone attacks can be the most painful of all medical emergencies.

Ten to twelve percent of the public will suffer at least one kidney stone attack at some point in their lives. Fortunately, many stones are tiny and smooth so they pass freely and are excreted without complications.

Kidney stone sufferers often lead sedentary lives or reside in dry (desert and mountain) and warm climates.

What To Look For

- A dull ache directly below the ribcage in the left or right mid-back, but not simultaneously on both sides.
- Left or right-sided backache, spreading forward to the lower abdomen and groin.
- Dark, rusty, or brownish urine. Blood in the urine is rare.
- Waves of sudden pain that stop for several minutes, then restart.
- Inability to find a comfortable position (in contrast to peritonitis where patients cannot move).
- Agitation. The patient can't get comfortable in any position so they move around and writhe in pain.

- Nausea, vomiting, and sweating.
- Fever and chills if the blockage creates a urinary tract or kidney infection (see Urinary Tract Disorders at p. 156).

What To Do
- Call 911.
- Have the patient drink as much water as possible, which may help them pass the stone. However, nausea and vomiting often make drinking fluids impossible.

What Not To Do
Do not give a patient painkillers until hospital testing is completed. Painkillers could disguise crucial symptoms and make diagnosis more difficult.

Typical Treatment
Hospital treatment centers on relieving pain and urinary tract blockage. Medications including morphine and Demerol® are injected for pain and intravenous fluids are given to flush out an obstructing stone.

Lower abdominal Xrays (KUB, for kidney-ureter-bladder) may reveal a white "pebble." A urinalysis may contain microscopic traces of blood.

Blood tests, including those to detect elevated white blood cell count, can disclose infections that require intravenous antibiotics and hospitalization. If Xrays do not reveal stones, additional tests may be ordered such as ultrasonography, CAT scans, or an IVP, an hour-long set of Xrays that reveals urinary tract blockage due to a stone that is "invisible." A patient will not be discharged until the stone has passed and the patient is infection free.

During hospitalization, all of the patient's urine in a twenty-four hour period is collected. This sample will be strained and the sediment retrieved will help identify the stone's constituents. There may be a high concentration of uric acid or abnormal excretion of calcium, citrate, and oxalate, any of which can cause kidney stones.

If a kidney stone does not pass within two to three days, the patient's kidneys will be bombarded with sound waves to pulverize the stone into tiny particles that can pass. If sonic bombardment fails, the stone can be surgically removed.

Follow-up Care

A patient should see a urologist within several days of hospital discharge, especially if the blockage caused an infection. The patient must continue to dilute his/her urine by drinking at least three liters of water each day. The patient may also be required to change his/her diet depending on the findings of the urine analyses. Possible changes include restricting salt, limiting protein, avoiding certain foods (for example rhubarb, cheese, or beer), and taking or avoiding calcium supplements.

Even after a change in diet and increase in fluid intake, kidney stone patients remain at risk for future attacks. Periodic twenty-four hour urine collections and radiological studies may be required to monitor whether new stones have formed. Patients can also check their urine at home for microscopic traces of blood by using test strips available at drugstores.

Dr. Fischer Says

Lower back pain on both sides of the spine is rarely, if ever, due to kidney stones.

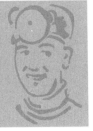

Marine Life Injuries

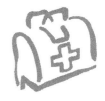

What They Are

Swimming in oceans and lakes can be treacherous. Besides drowning (see p. 68) and suffering diving injuries, patients can incur a wide range of life-threatening injuries from all sorts of marine life. For example, bites by sharks, barracuda, alligators, crocodiles, moray eels, sea snakes, and sea wasps are always medical emergencies. Shark, alligator, crocodile, and moray eel bites can tear through skin, crush and break and sever bones. Sea snake venom has more than double the toxicity of cobra venom and a sea wasp bite can kill a healthy patient in fifteen minutes.

Stings from jellyfish, Portuguese men of war, sponges, seaweed (limu), and sea anemone are usually less deadly. However, patients can suffer serious allergic reactions from the toxins released. For people with preexisting cardiac and respiratory conditions, these allergic reactions can be fatal.

Pinch wounds from crabs and lobsters and scratches, scrapes, and punctures from contact with coral, sea anemone, or sea urchin tentacles are usually minor irritants. However, when untreated they can cause nasty infections.

What to Look For
- Bleeding.
- Broken, crushed, or severed bones.
- Open puncture wounds, cuts, scratches, and scrapes.
- Labored or difficult breathing.
- Cold, clammy skin or sluggishness.

- Pain, red-hot rashes, muscle cramps, stomach pain, fever, chills, nausea, vomiting, labored breathing, and collapse (severe sting reactions, also known as anaphylaxis).
- Joint pain and swelling.
- Spines or tentacles.

What To Do

- Remove the patient from the water.
- Check whether the patient is breathing or has a pulse. If not, call 911 immediately and start CPR at once (see p. 173).
- Stop bleeding by applying gentle pressure on the wound with a clean cloth until the bleeding stops (see p. 181).
- If patient seems to be in shock (cold, clammy skin or sluggishness), elevate his/her feet and keep the patient warm and comfortable.
- Splint large wounds or broken limb bones (see p. 182).
- Find out what specific marine life caused the injury in order to assure that the patient gets the proper treatment.
- Cleanse closed wounds with antiseptic soap or seawater.
- Loosely bandage or apply sterile gauze pads to open wounds.
- Remove spines or tentacles left by marine creatures with the side of a sharp knife, tweezers, or tape. Soak the wound in hot water or a solution of either vinegar or rubbing alcohol and water for 15 to 30 minutes (until pain eases) and elevate the patient's feet.
- Keep sea snake victims as still as possible and follow the instructions for snake bites at p. 36.

What Not To Do

- Don't move the patient's head or neck if he/she is unconscious.
- Don't cut open a sea snake or sea wasp bite and try to suck out venom.

Typical Treatment

Large wounds will usually be cleaned and dead skin and foreign substances will be removed. Although large wounds are sutured, small wounds are usually left open, irrigated, and covered with sterile dressing. The patient will receive tetanus injections if they have not been immunized in the past five years. They will also be evaluated to see if they need minor surgery and/or antibiotics. The pain and discomfort from most sea stings is of short duration. However, when burning, itching, and warmness persist, the patient will be given topical antibiotics and tetanus toxoid injections. In the most serious cases of allergic reations (anaphylaxis), intravenous epinephrine injections will be given.

Follow-up Care

Wounds usually close without the need for suturing. They should be examined every two to three days to monitor the healing process and check for infection.

Dr. Fischer Says

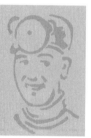

Although anthropological evidence suggests that man evolved from the sea (our cells have similar chemistry to sea water), we have always had an ambivalent relationship with creatures of deep and shallow waters. Always be aware of the possible dangers whenever you enter their realm!

Neck Injuries

What They Are

The spinal cord is a column filled with a network of delicate nerves. This network connects the brain to receptors, muscles, and organs throughout the body. Thirty-three bones called vertebrae protect the spinal cord. They sit one atop another and are connected by ligaments and separated by disks. In addition to protecting the spinal cord, the vertebrae support the chest and abdomen. As the spinal cord ascends towards the skull, it becomes more complex because it is joined by nerves from the legs, pelvis, abdomen, chest, and arms.

Injuries occur when the cervical spine, the seven vertebrae of the neck, is forced into twisted, over-flexed, over-extended, or other unnatural positions. Bones may fracture or dislocate and pinch, compress, or sever spinal nerves, which can cause severe pain, irreversible nerve damage, and paralysis. However, all cervical spine injuries don't necessarily produce immediate or permanent damage.

Osteoarthritis can involve the bones of the neck. However, slipped disks in the cervical neck area are rare.

Because of the complexity of the cervical spine, neck injuries may involve more nerve damage than lower spinal injuries. Furthermore, since the portion of the spine that supports the chest and abdomen is more rigid, trauma is usually transmitted to the flexible vertebrae in the neck. As a result, patients injured in car accidents often have "whiplash" injuries to the neck.

Patients with severe osteoporosis or bone cancer can suffer major injuries from relatively minor trauma. In the direst cases, cervical spine injuries can paralyze both arms, both legs, and the diaphragm and prevent patients from moving or breathing.

Car accidents, sports injuries, falls, and other trauma can also injure soft tissue structures (muscles, ligaments, tendons) and internal organs (trachea, digestive tract, or thyroid) of the neck.

Patients may feel stiffness and pain caused by swelling or bleeding in the neck muscles but appear normal to observers.

Bullet and knife wounds to the neck are extremely dangerous because they usually involve highly critical organs that are close to the surface. Stabbing and gunshot victims will need surgery once their heart and circulation have stabilized.

What To Look For
- Neck pain, tenderness, or stiffness, which often is felt hours later.
- Back, arm, or leg pain or stiffness.
- Paralysis of the arms, legs, or shoulders. Inability to move the toes.
- Numbness, tingling, or no feeling in the arms, legs, or shoulders.
- Shortness of breath (if the diaphragm or windpipe is affected).
- Nausea and vomiting.
- Hoarseness, difficulty swallowing, "laryngitis"-type speech (indicates damage to internal structures of the neck).

What To Do
- Call 911 immediately so that trained personnel can evaluate, stabilize, and transport the patient.
- After calling 911, keep the patient's neck and other affected areas motionless, even if the patient claims to be okay. *Immobility is the highest priority!* Since it is possible for people to walk with unstable spine fractures, don't allow patients to move.
- Support the patient's spine with small pieces of wood, heavy towels, sandbags, or a cervical collar, if available. Never move a patient's neck in order to support it or

move a twisted neck into the "correct position."

- Keep the patient lying flat. Patients with neck fractures may have very low blood pressure. If patients feel as if they're going to vomit, turn them and all supportive neck bracing to the side as a unit. This is called "log rolling" and requires at least two people working in close coordination. Failure to turn the patient may result in the patient's choking on vomit, which can be fatal.
- Check the patient's rate and depth of breathing. Neck injuries can paralyze the diaphragm, the muscle that facilitates breathing, and CPR may be needed (see p. 173).

What Not To Do

- Don't move a patient's neck in order to support it.
- Don't move, lift, or transport a neck or spinal injury patient by yourself.
- Don't allow a neck or spinal injury patient to stand or walk.

Typical Treatment

Emergency personnel will strap the patient to a transport board to protect against further injury. At the hospital, Xrays will be taken of all seven neck vertebrae and other injured areas. Neurological exams will be performed to look for spinal cord injuries that the initial Xrays might have missed. CT scans or MRIs may also be ordered to check that supportive structures were not injured.

In the hospital, the patient will be monitored for at least twenty-four hours even if tests didn't show fractures or spinal cord damage. If Xrays reveal fractures, traction devices will keep the bones from pressing on the spinal cord nerves.

Seriously injured patients will be admitted to a surgical intensive care unit and examined by orthopedists and neurosurgeons. If surgery is required, it may not be scheduled until after the patient's condition has stabilized, which usually takes several days. After surgery, patients will recuperate in a rehabilitation center for spinal-cord injury patients.

Blood pressure may plummet due to neck fractures (spinal shock). This will be relieved by slightly elevating the foot of the patient's bed. The patient's stomach will be emptied so the patient doesn't vomit and choke while lying on his back.

Follow-up Care

Patients who did not sustain fractures or dislocations should expect to experience considerable pain and stiffness for several days. Those who received soft tissue injuries will be given soft cervical collars for neck support. Ice packs applied during the first twenty-four hours may reduce tissue swelling.

Patients should be reexamined by an orthopedist about two or three days after discharge and, if full recovery isn't evident, about a week later. Mild muscle relaxants (Flexeril® or Robaxin®) or anti-inflammatory medications (Motrin® or Advil®) may help reduce their pain.

Dr. Fischer Says

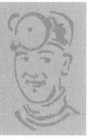

Because the risk of permanent damage is so great, anyone remotely suspected of a vertebral fracture should be assumed to have one until hospital testing is completed. Follow the Emergency Medicine adage: "A person who has neck pain after being touched by a feather has a cervical spine fracture until proved otherwise."

Nosebleeds

What They Are

Nosebleeds occur when blood vessels in our nasal passages rupture. They can strike without warning and be triggered by allergies, pollution, nose picking, overuse of nasal sprays, cold/dry weather, low humidity, and, of course, a punch in the nose. When arteries deep inside the nose break, often from hypertension and arteriosclerosis, blood can drain down the back of the throat and not be outwardly visible.

Patients who suffer from impaired blood clotting (hemophilia and other related blood diseases) are susceptible to nosebleeds. People who take aspirin, Coumadin®, or other blood thinners are also at risk. Offending medications should be discontinued, especially when arteries deep in the nasal cavity are damaged.

Since nosebleeds are common and usually stop within minutes, it is easy to minimize their significance. However, the blood loss from seemingly innocent nosebleeds can endanger elderly patients with poor circulation and heart problems. Persistent bleeding may cause them to choke on blood inhaled into their lungs.

What To Look For

- Bleeding from one nostril. Bleeding from both nostrils indicates a hemorrhage at the back of the nasal passages, an area that is inaccessible to pressure and cauterization.
- Pale, cold, and clammy skin signifying blood loss.
- Blood draining down the back of the throat, a dangerous sign.

Nosebleeds

What To Do

- If the bleeding is from both nostrils, call 911 immediately.
- If the bleeding is from one nostril, check for blood in the throat, which indicates deep, internal nasal bleeding.
- If the bleeding is internal, call 911 immediately. Internal nosebleeds cannot be treated at home or in a doctor's office.
- Keep the patient seated, head forward and facing downward, until arrival at a hospital.
- When the bleeding is from the front of the nose, apply cold compresses such as ice packs across the bridge of the nose that cover both sides.
- Pinch the nose for at least ten to fifteen minutes (as if you smelled a skunk).
- Allow the patient to sit slightly forward; never let the patient lie flat on his/her back.
- Get the patient to a hospital as soon as possible.

What Not To Do

- Don't let nosebleed patients touch or blow their noses. They could dislodge clots patching leaking vessels.
- Don't pack nostrils with cotton. It could cause blood to accumulate and flow down the throat.
- Don't let a nosebleed patient lie on his/her back since he/she could choke on blood.

Typical Treatment

First, medical personnel will take the patient's vital signs. Serious blood loss can lower blood pressure and accelerate the pulse rate. Patients with abnormal vital signs due to blood loss should be hospitalized for observation for twenty-four hours.

The bleeding area, if visible, will be inspected with specialized lamps, mirrors, and cauterizing tools. In most cases, the bleeding will have stopped and small scabs will be visible. Silver nitrate will be applied to control the bleeding. Epinephrine may be sprayed or swabbed on the area to constrict bleeding vessels. If bleeding continues, nasal tampons will be inserted and packed into the nostril to compress the injured vessel. Packing should remain in place for two to three days.

Bleeding from deep in the nasal passages requires hospitalization. This type of bleeding is usually more profuse and the damaged blood vessels are usually hard to see and cauterize. To seal bleeding vessels, emergency personnel will pack the nose, often using special nasal catheters (rubber tubes with small inflatable balloon tips filled with water). Catheters should remain in the nostrils until bleeding stops and patients' vital signs return to normal, which usually takes several days.

To prevent infection, patients will be put on antibiotics. Laboratory tests will monitor clotting time, platelet count, and assess the extent of the blood loss.

Follow-up Care

After two or three days, nasal packing is usually removed and further treatment is not required. Surgical repair (cauterization) of a nasal artery is rarely needed.

Patients should obtain information about and address medical and environmental conditions that might be causing their nosebleeds. They can include high blood pressure, anticoagulant medication, dust, or smog.

Dr. Fischer Says

Never underestimate nosebleeds and always err on the side of caution. Nosebleeds can be fatal. I once saw an otherwise healthy man die from nosebleed complications and a woman lose consciousness when her blood pressure dropped sharply. So, be on guard!

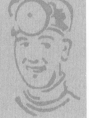

Pediatric Emergencies

What They Are

Children can be struck with virtually every type of medical emergency and diagnosis can be difficult because infants and small children can't describe what ails them. Pediatric emergencies can also be complicated by emotional factors such as fear, shyness, and lack of control. In addition, a particular symptom may not indicate the actual problem and the child may simply be lethargic, irritable, or not hungry.

Therefore, when you notice behavioral changes, fever, rashes, or pain, immediately notify the family pediatrician. ER physicians handle over thirty million pediatric cases each year, so erring on the side of caution is always advisable.

What To Look For

Intestinal Colic
- Children under six months old.
- Episodes of crying for several hours. The infant may be suffering from too much air in the intestines, hunger, or dehydration.

Apnea
- No breathing.
- Unresponsiveness.
- Turning blue.

Infectious Mononucleosis ("kissing disease")
- Red, sore throat and difficulty swallowing. May resemble a "strep throat."
- Swollen neck glands.

- Yellow skin color (jaundice), abdominal pain, and nausea may indicate enlargement of the spleen and liver (hepatitis).

Sickle-Cell Disease
- Severe pain anywhere in the body, but usually in the abdomen or limbs. Blood clots may form in small arteries, usually triggered by infection, dehydration, or stress.
- Prevalent in African-Americans usually in an inactive form (sickle-cell trait).

Skin Rashes Due to Infectious Diseases
- Red, pink, or white spots.
  - Measles—Red spots first appear behind the ears.
  - Rubella—Red spots first appear on face and neck.
  - Chickenpox—Clear spots first appear on the trunk.
  - Rocky Mountain spotted fever—Red spots appear on the hands and feet a few days after a tick bite.
- Yellow bumps filled with pus, scaling, and crusting of the lips, face, and limbs are signs of impetigo, which is highly contagious.

Epiglottis/croup
- Swelling and narrowing of the upper airways.
- Difficulty breathing due to airflow obstruction.
- A high-pitched noise or wheeze when inhaling (stridor).
- Fever.
- "Scratchy" voice.
- Difficulty swallowing.
- Coughing or drooling.
- **NOTE:** Choking on objects (food or toys) has similar signs, except for fever.

Pediatric Emergencies

Abdominal Pain
- A severe, diffuse, continuous abdominal pain that worsens with movement may indicate ruptured appendicitis and peritonitis.
- Pain occurring and disappearing in waves. May be due to structural or mechanical abnormalities of the intestines such as twisting (volvulus), telescoping (intussuseption), or herniation (into the groin or umbilicus).

Febrile Seizures
- Rapid elevation of temperature.
- Sudden shaking of the entire body.
- Return to normal level of consciousness (unlike epilepsy).

Bronchiolitis
- Severe difficulty breathing.
- Wheezing (bronchiolitis may be a precursor to asthma).
- Runny nose.

Meningitis
- Fever and listlessness.
- Poor appetite, nausea, and vomiting.
- Sensitivity to bright light.
- Neck stiffness.
- Possible seizures.

What To Do

Infants or children with any of the above conditions need immediate medical attention. If you suspect intestinal colic, mononucleosis, or if the child has a rash, call a pediatrician. Otherwise:

- Call 911 immediately.

Pediatric Emergencies

- Comfort and carefully watch the child.
- Perform CPR if the child stops breathing (see p. 173).
- Perform the Heimlich Maneuver if the child is choking.

Intestinal Colic
Burp and comfort the infant, but it may not bring relief. When in doubt, call a pediatrician.

Apnea
Call 911 immediately and begin CPR to restore the child's circulation.

Infectious Mononucleosis
Call your pediatrician. Give the child bed rest and fluids and keep the child away from other children. Expect two or more weeks for recovery.

Sickle Cell Disease
Call 911 immediately. A sickle cell crisis cannot be treated at home and requires inpatient hospital care.

Skin Rashes: measles, rubella and chickenpox
Call a pediatrician—who may direct you to give the child Tylenol® and fluids.

Impetigo
Call a pediatrician—who may prescribe antibiotics. Carefully cleanse the skin.

Epiglottis/croup
Call 911 immediately. The child will need hospital treatment to open constricted air passageways.

Perforated Appendicitis
Call 911 immediately because the patient will require prompt surgery.

Febrile Seizures

Call 911 immediately. ER evaluation is needed to ascertain the cause of the fever and to make sure that the child does not have epilepsy or meningitis. Stay calm; children snap out of febrile seizures once their temperatures go down.

Bronchiolitis

Call 911 immediately. Emergency personnel will give the child oxygen and may start intravenous fluids.

Meningitis

Call 911 immediately. Emergency personnel will give the child oxygen and may start intravenous fluids.

What Not To Do

- Don't give food or water to children who have abdominal pain, signs of meningitis, or breathing difficulties.
- Don't give children Tylenol® or antibiotics; they may mask symptoms and make diagnosis more difficult. Always avoid giving children aspirin.

Typical Treatment

Intestinal Colic

There is no known medical treatment for this condition, and it may need to be distinguished from life-threatening abdominal emergencies by the pediatrician or ER staff.

Apnea

The ER staff will monitor and usually hospitalize all infants and children whose breathing may have stopped. Blood tests, Xrays, EKGs, and other diagnostic tests may be ordered.

Infectious Mononucleosis

There is no antibiotic treatment for this viral illness and recuperation may take several weeks. Patients will be monitored for signs of complications such as hepatitis and rupture of the spleen.

Sickle Cell Disease
Treatment may include pain medication, oxygen, intravenous fluids, and possibly transfusions. A blood test can identify this genetically transmitted disease.

Skin Rashes
After a few days of bed rest, measles, rubella, and chickenpox usually pass without complications. Patients with impetigo and Rocky Mountain spotted fever will be given oral antibiotics.

Epiglottis/croup
ER staff will provide oxygen, epinephrine, intravenous steroids, and possibly antibiotics. Children who become lethargic or unable to breathe effectively may need mechanical ventilation or a tracheotomy. Choking on foreign objects can resemble croup. If present, small inhaled items (beans, eraser tips, peas) may have to be removed under general anesthesia.

Perforated Appendicitis
Immediate surgery is needed when appendicitis is complicated by peritonitis.

Febrile Seizures
ER staff must locate the site of infection and may need to extract spinal fluid. Unlike epilepsy, there is no disorientation or confusion after the seizure. Treatment of the cause of fever (with Tylenol® and or antibiotics) is of prime importance. Antiepilepsy medication is usually not needed. Children usually suffer no damage and outgrow this condition.

Bronchiolitis
Medication is given to open narrowed lung passages and patients will also receive

oxygen, acetaminophen, and intravenous fluids. In severe cases, hospitalization and/or mechanical ventilation may be necessary.

Meningitis

ER evaluation is needed immediately. Meningitis is a major medical emergency and patients will need intravenous antibiotics as soon as possible. Children who have been exposed to meningitis will need immediate medical evaluation and will usually be given oral antibiotics as a precautionary measure.

Follow-up Care

Children are amazingly resilient and most recover from pediatric emergencies without permanent complications or developmental problems. However, all patients should see a pediatrician several days after they were treated in the ER or hospitalized.

Make sure that children do not sleep face down. In this position, they may retain excessive carbon dioxide. Sudden Infant Death Syndrome is a mysterious and thus far poorly understood calamity of sudden respiratory arrest.

Dr. Fischer Says

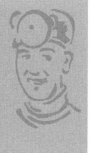

No one goes through childhood without several, hopefully minor, medical emergencies. Regular pediatric checkups and good communication between parents and doctors decreases the possibility of serious problems and complications.

As a child, I contracted scarlet fever, a bacterial infection that resembles tonsillitis. My pediatrician recognized the raised red rash all over my body and my bright, strawberry-red tongue and gave me penicillin, which is still the accepted treatment for scarlet fever.

133

Phlebitis

What It Is

Phlebitis is a condition in which blood clots (thrombi) form inside blood vessels. Although these clots can form in any blood vessel, they appear most commonly in the veins of women's legs. Phlebitis strikes pregnant women, women on oral contraceptives, bedridden and postoperative patients, as well as the obese, smokers, the elderly, and those with varicose veins. Large blood clots can also block the arteries of patients with severe "hardening of the arteries" and atrial fibrillation. Patients develop sudden pain in an arm or leg, which becomes pale, cold, numb, or paralyzed.

Phlebitis can be excruciatingly painful. However, superficial phlebitis, which affects veins visible on the legs' surface, is usually not life-threatening. When phlebitis is deep in hidden calf veins, it can be dangerous. Small pieces of a clot can break off, enter the bloodstream, and block tiny arteries in the lungs. This can cut off circulation, injure the lung, and block the normal exchange of oxygen and carbon dioxide (acute pulmonary embolism).

What To Look For

- Redness, swelling, warmth, and tenderness in the affected area. Inflamed veins may appear near the surface of the leg.
- A pale, cold, numb, or paralyzed limb (an acute arterial occlusion due to atrial fibrillation).
- Severe pain and swelling in the back of the lower leg, which often intensifies when standing or walking.

Phlebitis

- Calf pain when moving the foot of the affected leg up and down.
- If patients with calf pain were recently confined to bed rest or were seated for prolonged periods (in airplanes, for example), assume that they might have phlebitis.
- Sudden shortness of breath, palpitations, chest pains, and heart rhythm disturbances (acute pulmonary embolism).
- You may not be able to see or feel a clotted varicose vein.

What To Do
- Place the patient flat on his/her back.
- Elevate the leg until the affected vein is higher than the heart, unless the leg is pale, cold, and numb.
- Place a warm compress on the inflamed, tender area, for example, a towel moistened with tap water.
- If the pain is severe call 911 and notify the patient's doctor.

What Not To Do
Do not allow patients to sit, stand, or walk.

Typical Treatment
Blood tests, EKGs, or Xrays cannot confirm whether the patient has phlebitis. Therefore, the diagnosis is made primarily from the patient's history and from a physical examination. However, a Doppler sonogram is often helpful.

Anticoagulants such as low-molecular weight heparin can be injected into the skin to thin the blood, inhibit clot growth and prevent clot fragments from traveling to the lungs. Usually, Coumadin®, an oral anticoagulant, is given along with heparin for the first two to three days.

Patients receiving the stronger anticoagulants (for deep phlebitis) must be monitored for possible hemorrhaging unrelated to phlebitis, including bleeding stomach ulcers or blood in the urine.

Phlebitis

Thanks to our coagulation system, blockages usually improve in about six to eight hours and clots in lung arteries (pulmonary emboli) become less likely.

Follow-up Care

Hospitalization usually lasts for several days as swelling, pain, and redness disappear.

After discharge, patients will remain on oral anticoagulants, such as Coumadin®, for several months to prevent further clotting. Elastic stockings that gently support the calf muscles also help the circulation, but other tight, constricting leg wear can be dangerous. Conditions that contribute to phlebitis such as inactivity, obesity, and use of oral contraceptives must also be addressed.

Dr. Fischer Says

Proceed gently when elevating a patient's leg above the heart or when moving the patient's leg in any other way. Never squeeze or touch the affected area because you might cause a clot, or a piece of a clot, to break free and travel to the patient's lungs!

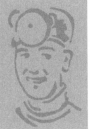

Pneumonia

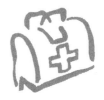

What It Is

When infectious agents such as bacteria and viruses are inhaled, they can overwhelm the lungs' defense mechanisms and flood the lungs with secretions. This impairs the exchange of oxygen and carbon dioxide and causes shortness of breath, extreme weakness, and often delirium.

Pneumonia is the sixth leading cause of death in the U.S.A. The infection may be more severe for patients confined to nursing homes, as well as those suffering from emphysema, diabetes, chronic alcoholism, and receiving chemotheraphy for cancer.

"Walking pneumonia" is the condition where patients with pneumonia don't exhibit signs or symptoms of the disease. Unrecognized and untreated lung infections can be life-threatening.

Pleuritis is the inflammation or infection of the membranes that line the lungs. It can be fatal. When severe, pleuritis can limit the lungs' ability to expand and inflate. This may allow bacteria to enter the bloodstream where they multiply and release toxins (septicemia) that can cause a dangerous drop in the patient's blood pressure.

Acute bronchitis is a milder infection than pneumonia and is usually confined to the upper airways, not the lungs. Patients will have fever, muscle aches, and runny nose, but none of the more dramatic symptoms.

What To Look For

- Shortness of breath.
- Rapid breathing. A pulse over 120 indicates a severe emergency.

Pneumonia

- Severe coughing.
- Gurgling sounds when breathing.
- Green, yellow, bloody, or rusty phlegm.
- Muscle and joint pain.
- Severe fatigue, weakness, or dizziness.
- Fever.
- Chills (uncontrollable shaking).
- Blue lips or fingertips.
- Appetite loss.
- Delirium or confusion.
- Pneumonia may have no clear-cut respiratory signs. So look for uncharacteristic irritability and restlessness in the very young and loss of appetite in the elderly.

What To Do

- Call 911 immediately if the patient appears dehydrated, disoriented, extremely weak, or unable to drink.
- Take the patient for emergency treatment if he/she is breathing rapidly (more than 20 breaths per minute), making "gurgling" sounds, has blue lips or fingertips, a severe cough, or uncontrollable chills.
- Notify the patient's doctor, if possible. Pneumonia can be diagnosed in the doctor's office, but patients who appear very ill may need emergency room evaluation.
- Keep the patient warm, at rest, and seated if possible (to avoid choking).
- Apply warm, moist compresses to the chest.
- Give the patient Tylenol®, aspirin, or supplemental oxygen, if available.
- For bronchitis, call the patient's doctor and follow the instructions given.

What Not To Do

- Don't allow the patient to minimize his/her condition by suggesting, "It's only the flu."
- Don't let the patient use other people's antibiotics because they may undermine laboratory tests.

Typical Treatment

A chest Xray will usually reveal the presence of pneumonia. Blood tests will determine the severity of the infection and degree of repiratory impairment. Oxygen and intravenous fluids are administered to stabilize the patient's vital signs and circulation.

When tests identify offending bacteria (viruses cannot be cultured or seen under the usual microscopes), antibiotics are given. Antibiotics will be started as soon as bacteria coughed up in a sputum sample have been identified under a microscope.

When infections are life-threatening, two intravenous antibiotics are immediately given to prevent septicemia. They are often started before the test results are available.

Although hospital confinement is usually preferred for seriously ill patients, the emergency room staff will decide whether to admit a patient or send him/her home on oral antibiotics. Medications prescribed include penicillin, Bactrim®, erythromycin, Cipro®, and doxycycline.

A patient with pneumonia that affects both lungs or that produces large amounts of respiratory secretions is monitored in the intensive care unit. Bed rest and a proper diet (either at home or in the hospital) are required for the patient's recovery.

Follow-up Care

Expect improvement to take at least a week. Improvement can take longer with patients who also suffer from conditions such as diabetes, emphysema, cystic fibrosis, asthma, and coronary disease. A patient should continue taking antibiotics until the fever, white cell elevation, high respiratory rate, and cough are under control.

Dr. Fischer Says

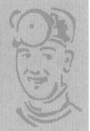

Practice counting respiration rates so that you can tell if patients' breathing is impaired. Watch and count the chest expansions of your family and friends. The normal rate is eighteen breaths per minute. If you suspect pneumonia, look for shaking chills—the most ominous sign of the condition and if they are present, get emergency help!

Poisoning and Drug Abuse

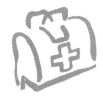

What They Are

Adverse physical or mental reactions can occur when we ingest, inhale, or touch toxic substances...solid, liquid, or gas. These toxins can destroy organs, cells, and tissues and prevent our systems from functioning properly. The damage can be immediate, delayed, or both and may or may not have characteristic signs or symptoms.

Antidotes exist for some poisons, but not all. In the absence of antidotes, critically ill patients will be connected to machines that breathe for them (mechanical ventilators) and monitored in an intensive care unit until the poison is metabolized, neutralized, and excreted.

Carbon monoxide, cocaine, and tricyclic antidepressants are the most deadly toxic substances. Then come acetaminophen, tranquilizers, lead, and opiates (primarily heroin).

Recreational drugs can be lethal—especially when several drugs are taken together, for example, alcohol, sedatives, and stimulants. Only hospitals are equipped to handle these complex emergencies.

Other medical emergencies caused by specific poisons include seizures, heart-rhythm disturbances, breathing disorders, coma, hyperthermia (extremely high body temperature) and blood-chemistry imbalances. Since dangerous chemicals remain in the bloodstream for hours, patients can develop any of these life-threatening conditions when the toxins are in their systems.

What To Look For

• Incoherent speech.

- Small pupils or extremely wide pupils.
- Blue lips or fingertips.
- Stumbling while walking.
- Shallow breathing.
- Disorientation.
- Seizures.
- Signs of an apparent suicide attempt.

What To Do

- For drug overdoses or severe poisonings, call 911 immediately. Time is of the essence—a life could be in danger!
- When in doubt, promptly call 911. It is often impossible to know how much poison a patient has absorbed. So, always err on the side of caution because a patient's respiratory rate or blood pressure can drop suddenly.
- A patient who has swallowed milder poisons (such as pills) should drink syrup of ipecac. Ipecac will cause vomiting, which expels toxins that have not yet been absorbed in the bloodstream. *Do not give syrup of ipecac to patients who swallowed caustic substances such as lye or to those having epileptic seizures.*
- If a patient inhales and collapses from noxious chemicals (smoke or chemical emissions), remove the patient from exposure. Call 911 immediately and try to provide fresh air until emergency personnel arrive.
- Place the patient on one side until emergency personnel arrive to eliminate the danger of choking on vomit.

What Not To Do

- Don't give syrup of ipecac to patients who have taken caustic substances such as lye. Although lye is dangerous, it should be left in the stomach where it will be neutralized by acid. Vomiting lye might severely burn the esophagus.

• Don't induce vomiting or give syrup of ipecac to sleepy or lethargic patients or patients having epileptic seizures. They could become nauseated and choke on their vomit.

Typical Treatment

Treatment will initially focus on stabilizing the patient's vital signs; cardiac monitoring and respiratory support will be the top priorities. Poisonous substances will then be removed or neutralized and intravenous fluids will be administered to normalize blood pressure and speed the metabolism of toxins.

A tube will be inserted through the patient's mouth or nose into his/her stomach. The contents of the patient's stomach will be flushed out with sterile water. Then the patient will be given activated charcoal to bind potentially toxic chemicals before they pass from the intestines to the bloodstream.

A patient who overdoses on street drugs will receive naloxone (Narcan®), the antidote for opiate intoxication. Naloxone immediately reverses heroin, morphine, codeine, or methadone overdoses and may cause withdrawal, which in itself can be a medical emergency.

Other specific poison remedies include high doses of oxygen for carbon monoxide, dialysis for medications such as lithium or acid/base imbalances, chelation for lead and mercury, amyl nitrite for cyanide, atropine for insecticide, methylene blue for nitrogenous compounds, physostigmine for antidepressants, and NAC for acetaminophcn.

When the cause of poisoning or an overdose is unknown, the patient's stomach will be washed out. The patient will be given activated charcoal, antiopiate medication, and supportive care (such as mechanical ventilation and monitoring in an intensive care unit). Chest Xrays will check for accidental inhalation of stomach contents.

Patients who took or were exposed to dangerous toxins that metabolize slowly will remain hospitalized, often in the intensive care unit, where they will be monitored and treated.

Follow-up Care

After patients are discharged from the ER, their family and friends should closely monitor their behavior. Patients who overdosed on either recreational drugs or as a result of suicide attempts will undergo psychological evaluation before they are discharged.

After discharge, they should continue counseling.

Dr. Fischer Says

Treat every poisoning and drug overdose as life-threatening. Don't delay calling 911. While you are waiting for help to arrive, place the patient on one side to prevent choking if vomiting occurs.

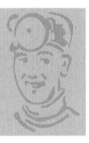

Seizures

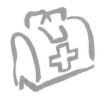

What They Are

Seizures are uncontrollable, severe, spasmodic body movements (jerking) that are accompanied by altered levels of consciousness. Seizures are also known as epileptic seizures or convulsions. Epilepsy, a major cause of seizures, is a hereditary condition of unknown origin that begins in childhood or adolescence and can last a lifetime.

Seizures fall into several classifications. Generalized seizures (greand mal epilepsy) are the most dramatic because patients lose consciousness, fall to the ground, and their bodies shake with convulsions. Convulsions often alternate with the spastic extension of all four limbs. Seizure attacks usually last one to two minutes and are often followed by loss of bladder control.

During a seizure, a patient may bite the tongue, fracture or dislocate bones, or inhale vomit or respiratory secretions. Therefore, prompt emergency medical care should be sought, especially if the seizures are continuous or recur during a thirty-minute period and the patient does not regain consciousness.

When a seizure ends, patients are usually in a stupor for ten to twenty minutes, followed by twenty to thirty minutes of extreme confusion and disorientation.

Absence seizures (petit mal epilepsy) usually last only a few seconds. Patients typically stare blankly while their eyelids blink. They don't collapse or shake with convulsions. When they regain consciousness, they have no memory of the seizure.

Partial seizures are due to abnormal electrical discharges in one area of the brain. Patients usually experience a specific physical reaction, principally twitching of a single body part such as one arm or leg.

Seizures

Partial and petit mal seizures are less life-threatening than generalized or grand mal seizures. However, after their initial episode, all patients should get emergency treatment as soon as possible.

Seizures occurring after a head injury are called secondary or post-traumatic epilepsy. Seizures can also be caused by high fever, sedative or alcohol withdrawal, sleep deprivation, stress, or abuse of stimulants. See Obstetric Disorders at p. 164 for a discussion of Eclampsia, a syndrome of seizures, high blood pressure, and edema that strikes pregnant women.

What To Look For
- Convulsions (erratic bodily jerking).
- Loss of consciousness.
- Stretching or extending all four limbs.
- Loss of bladder control.
- Confusion and disorientation.
- Flashing lights, strange smells, "pins and needles" tingling that lasts twenty to thirty seconds (unusual premonitions called "auras" are experienced by some patients).

What To Do
- Call 911, but don't leave a patient alone during a seizure, even to call 911. Make sure the patient's condition has stabilized before calling 911.
- Get the patient off his/her feet so he/she can't fall.
- Turn the patient on his/her side to prevent choking on gastric or respiratory secretions (or blood, if the tongue is accidentally bitten).

What Not To Do
- Don't leave the patient unattended during a seizure, even to call 911.
- Don't allow the patient to fall.

- Don't push anything into the patient's mouth. It might push the patient's tongue further back and cause him/her to choke.

Typical Treatment

Hospitalization for twenty-four-hour observation is usually needed for first-time sufferers. Patients who had seizures due to head injuries and pregnant woman with eclampsia are always admitted for observation and treatment. Patients with chronic epilepsy may be discharged if they recover quickly and did not sustain any significant physical injuries.

A seizure patient receives intravenous medication such as Valium®, Dilantin®, or phenobarbital to stabilize his/her condition. Patients are given tests that aid in diagnosis including MRIs or CT scans, electroencephalograms, and lumbar punctures. Unfortunately, some test results may be deceptively normal between seizures.

Follow-up Care

The patient's physician or consulting neurologist will decide whether to put the patient on daily antiepileptic medication such as Dilantin®, carbamazepine, and vaproic acid. Although many antiepileptic drugs exist, they all have side effects. Medication taken regularly usually stops most seizures, but many patients on medication still have "breakthrough" seizures.

Social and psychological factors such as stress, fatigue, embarrassment, and discrimination should be addressed. By understanding the nature of their condition and epilepsy itself, patients and their families can handle it more effectively.

Dr. Fischer Says

Many epileptics sense the onset of an attack. Despite the dramatic nature of epilepsy, seizures don't directly traumatize the brain or the body. Patients usually return to normal after about an hour of sleepiness and confusion.

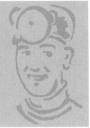

Skin Emergencies and Allergies

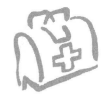

What They Are

When we come in contact with certain toxic substances, our skin acts as our bodies' first line of defense. It warns us of danger by breaking out in lesions, hives, bumps, and blotches and by making us tear, sniffle, or itch. These signals are hard to ignore, but it is surprising how many people pay them no heed.

Rashes and skin eruptions account for about five percent of adult and thirty percent of pediatric ER visits. Drug, food, and other allergies are among the most common causes of skin emergencies. Often, they are the first warning to steer clear of shellfish, peanuts, penicillin, cats, wool, and other irritants. Other substances that trigger allergic reactions include aspirin, milk, eggs, sulfa drugs, iodine contrast dyes, mismatched blood transfusions, wasp, bee, and ant stings, and poison ivy, oak, and sumac. When sensitive patients come in contact with these items, they can get severe allergic reactions that, if not promptly treated, can be life-threatening.

Shingles is a reactivation of chicken pox virus in adults that affects the nerves of the trunk, face, or eye on one side. Shingles produces an extremely painful rash but is not contagious.

Sunburn is a severe first-degree burn due to prolonged exposure to ultraviolet light (see Burns, at p. 47).

What To Look For

- Bumps on the skin, either clear "hives," or reddened rashes.
- Complaints that "my entire body is hot" or "itchy."

Skin Emergencies and Allergies

- Swelling of the face, neck, or tongue.
- Hives or other lesions in the mouth may be signs of impending upper airway constriction. Additional signs are patients sounding hoarse, coughing, and developing shortness of breath.
- Ask:
  - Where is the rash? Is it localized to one part of the body or everywhere?
  - Did it occur suddenly or gradually?
  - Does it hurt, itch, or neither?
  - Did it become apparent after exposure or contact with food, drugs, or plants?
  - Did the rash appear after exposure to sunlight?
  - What color is the rash?
  - How old is the patient? (To rule out measles or chicken pox.)
  - Is the patient on prescription medication?
- Skin lesions all over the body could indicate dangerous infectious diseases such as syphilis, gonorrhea, meningitis, or Rocky Mountain spotted fever.
- A small, itchy rash on a single body part usually indicates a localized allergic reaction (contact dermatitis) that was activated by touching an irritant such as fabrics, plants, jewelry, hair products, or cosmetics.
- Small clusters of tiny "bubbles" may be poison ivy/oak/sumac, which can itch like crazy and spread like wildfire.
- Extremely painful clusters of "bubbles" on one side of the torso or face may be shingles.
- Redness, blistering, and pain after prolonged exposure to the sun is usually sunburn.

What To Do
- Call 911 immediately if the patient has hives or rashes in the mouth. Speed is of the essence since the patient's breathing passages could constrict.

- Call 911 if the patient has swelling of the face, neck, lips, or tongue (angioedema).
- Call 911 immediately if the patient sounds hoarse or is short of breath. The patient's blood pressure could plummet and the patient may collapse (anaphylactic shock).
- Call 911 immediately if the patient has a rash all over his/her body, fever, malaise, headache, vomiting, or neck stiffness (meningitis or Rocky Mountain spotted fever).
- Rush children with rashes to a pediatrician (or pediatric ER). Their problem could be relatively harmless (chicken pox or measles) or extremely serious (meningitis).

What Not To Do

- Don't allow the patient to minimize his/her symptoms, especially if you see the rash worsen in front of your eyes.
- Don't attempt to diagnose a child's condition. Just rush him/her to a pediatrician.

Typical Treatment

Small, itchy rashes due to localized allergic reactions are usually treated with over-the-counter steroid creams. Superficial infections and abscesses generally respond to topical or oral antibiotics or draining. Infection of the deeper tissue layers (cellulitis) is normally treated with intravenous antibiotics and may necessitate hospitalization.

Poison ivy/oak patients usually receive steroid pills for two or three days starting as soon as possible.

Emergency facilities treat allergic reactions with antihistamines such as Benadryl®, and injections of adrenalinelike medication (epinephrine). A patient suspected of having upper airway obstruction may be hospitalized because, even if he/she initially improves, potentially fatal toxins may remain in the bloodstream. The most serious cases may be given intravenous epinephrine, antihistamines, or steroids and receive mechanical support for breathing.

For shingles, acyclovir pills are prescribed for one week.

WARNING: If you treat an allergic reaction at home with Benadryl®, follow up with an examination or a phone call to your physician as soon as possible.

Follow-up Care

Patients will be discharged from ERs when their intense initial itching, warmness, and redness begin to subside, which usually takes three to four hours. They should continue taking antihistamines for another day or two.

Skin rashes can last for at least a week, long after the toxic trigger has left the body. Patients should be reassured that his/her appearance won't be affected since cosmetic damage seldom occurs.

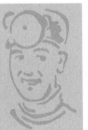

Dr. Fischer Says

Second or subsequent reactions often increase in intensity and can result in a catastrophic drop of blood pressure (anaphylactic shock). If you have had an allergic reaction, find out what caused it and eliminate it from your life. Keep Benadryl® 25 mg. tablets at home, which can be bought without a prescription.

Strokes

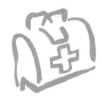

What They Are

Strokes are the third leading cause of deaths in the U.S.A.; over 700,000 occur yearly. They can permanently paralyze patients and make them unable to care for themselves. Strokes are caused by blood clots (thrombi) or large pieces of cholesterol plaque that block arteries and cut off the circulation of oxygen to the brain. When nerve cells are deprived of oxygen, they die in a few minutes.

Emboli (pieces of blood clots) cause blockages when they travel downstream from either the heart walls or the inner surface of the large carotid arteries in the neck.

Extremely high blood pressure, usually 220/120 or more, may cause blood vessels to break and bleed directly into brain tissue (hemorrhagic stroke).

Aneurysms are small weak areas in the cerebral arterial walls that may swell, burst, and flood the brain with blood.

A stroke affecting the breathing center of the brain can cause a heart attack and, conversely, strokes can be triggered by heart attacks.

TIA (transient ischemic attack) is a temporary neurological impairment caused by a blocked cerebral artery. If not immediately treated, it can cause permanent damage. TIAs last less than twenty-four hours and about eighty percent of cases resolve within thirty minutes.

What To Look For

- Inability to move, stand, talk, or communicate. A patient may be unable to answer simple questions or identify family members.

- Paralysis. Usually, only one side of the body is affected. For example, a patient with a clot on the left side of the brain (that affects the speech and motor areas) cannot move the right side of his/her body and cannot talk.
- Severe headache.
- Double vision.
- Dizziness.
- Nausea and vomiting.

What To Do

- Call 911 immediately. Prompt action can truly be a matter of life or death.
- Call 911 immediately if the patient is a diabetic. Hypoglycemia due to an insulin reaction may look exactly like a stroke.
- Check whether the patient is breathing and has a pulse. If not, begin CPR (see CPR at p. 173).
- If a patient is nauseous or vomiting, tilt the head or body slightly to one side.
- Keep an alert patient resting comfortably because balance and ability to bear weight may be impaired.

What Not To Do

Don't give aspirin and similar pain relievers to patients with severe headache and nausea. Aspirin is a blood thinner that could exacerbate strokes caused by bleeding into the brain. Stronger painkillers may have a sedating effect on patients, which can also be dangerous.

Typical Treatment

Initially, emergency personnel will try to stabilize the patient's heart and breathing functions by giving oxygen, intravenous fluids, and antihypertensive medication, when appropriate. When a patient is stabilized, CAT scans will determine if an area of the brain did not receive blood or blood flooded and compressed brain tissue.

Strokes

A patient having a stroke caused by the blockage of a narrow, arteriosclerotic artery may receive blood thinners, such as heparin, Coumadin®, aspirin, or tPA (a new treatment that must be given within six hours of the stroke). TPA is an intravenous medication that helps dissolve clots and restore blood flow. However, a patient with documented bleeding into the brain cannot receive any blood thinners. A consulting neurologist will decide which medications are appropriate.

EKGs will check for heart damage and rhythm disturbances. Chest Xrays will be taken to detect pneumonia. Echocardiograms may reveal clots on the inner surface of the heart (a potential source of emboli).

Follow-up Care

Patients, including those with TIAs, must continue to be hospitalized. The extent of their neurological damage will be assessed and their condition will be monitored. Other necessary tests may include carotid sonography and cerebral angiograms. Blockages found in neck arteries can sometimes be removed by a surgical procedure (carotid endarterectomy).

When the acute illness passes, physical rehabilitation and psychological support will begin, which can be a long, arduous road.

Patients who are unable to care for themselves must have full-time in-home care or be placed in nursing homes.

Dr. Fischer Says

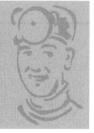

Always check a suspected stroke patient's pulse and breathing! Stroke victims often run a high risk for other clot-related illnesses such as heart attacks. Place patients slightly to one side, not flat on their backs, so they don't choke on gastric or respiratory secretions.

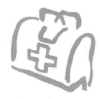

Urinary Tract Disorders

What They Are

Medical problems can occur along the path that urine travels after it forms in the kidneys. These problems can be infections or dysfunctions of the kidneys, the ureter (the tube that carries urine to the bladder), the bladder (the organ that stores urine until it's expelled), and the urethra (the opening through which urine exits the body).

Men may also suffer from swelling or infection of the prostate gland, a walnut-sized organ that can enlarge and compress the urethra. Untreated urinary tract infections may develop into life-threatening kidney infections.

Urine rarely contains harmful amounts of bacteria because of its acid chemistry. However, when the outflow is partially blocked by an enlarged prostate, a pregnancy, or a kidney stone, bacteria can multiply in the stagnant urinary system. *E. coli*, pathogens normally found in the large intestine, are the most common culprit. Women are more prone to urinary tract infections than men because of the proximity of their urethra to external bacteria.

Acute urinary retention occurs when the urinary path is suddenly blocked. Men over age 60 may get this painful condition when the prostate gland enlarges and prevents the bladder from emptying properly. If urine and bacteria back up into the kidneys and/or bloodstream (*urosepsis*), it can cause shock or death.

What To Look For

Bladder Infections (cystitis)

• Burning sensation during urination.
• A dramatic increase in urinary frequency (often hourly).

- Pain in the central lower abdomen (the bladder area).
- Fever.
- Blood in the urine.

Kidney Infections (pyelonephritis)
- The symptoms listed above plus:
- Severe pain on one side of the lower back (flank pain).
- Nausea, vomiting, and shaking chills.

Urinary Retention
- Pain and swelling over the central lower abdomen (bladder).

What To Do
- When a urinary tract infection is suspected, immediately call the patient's physician.
- When the patient has chills, vomiting, and/or flank pain, immediately call 911.
- If urine is being retained (pain over the bladder), immediately call 911.

What Not To Do
- Don't delay calling 911 if urinary retention or acute kidney infections are even remotely suspected.
- Don't give a patient another person's antibiotics. Those medicines may be ineffective or harmful and may complicate proper diagnosis.

Typical Treatment
The patient's history, vital signs, and physical examination will determine the severity of his/her condition. Blood and urine tests will confirm whether the patient has a bladder infection. A urine culture will be taken to identify the presence of specific bacteria and to determine which antibiotics are most effective. An extremely ill patient will have blood cultured to see if actively multiplying bacteria have entered the circulatory system. Antibiotics are often given before the results are available.

Urinary Tract Disorders

Emergency patients with acute urinary retention may need a bladder catheterization. In this procedure, a physician inserts a thin, sterile, rubber tube into the urinary tract. The tube opens a pathway and allows urine to drain from the bladder. The urine expelled will be examined for signs of infection.

Patients with kidney infections, urinary blockage, or sepsis (bacteria in the bloodstream) will usually be hospitalized and given intravenous fluids and antibiotics such as Cipro®. Expect hospitalization to last for at least a week. Consultations by a urologist and diagnostic Xray tests should determine the correct diagnosis and course of treatment.

When men under age fifty have symptoms such as burning upon urination and discharge from the penis, they are usually due to sexually transmitted diseases such as gonorrhea and chlamydia. These men are placed on a regimen of antibiotics including penicillin, amoxicillin, Flagyl®, and Rocephin® and their sexual partners are examined to prevent further spread of these diseases.

Follow-up Care

Most patients with uncomplicated urinary tract infections receive oral antibiotics (Bactrim®, Macrodantin®, or Cipro®) and are sent home. They should see their physician a few days after ER discharge. Patients should continue taking medication for three to ten days as directed by their physician, at which time their urine will be reexamined and recultured to determine if all infectious agents have disappeared.

Patients with more complex problems will continue to be monitored by their physicians.

Dr. Fischer Says

Urinary tract infections account for over six million medical office visits every year and two thirds of the patients are women. Painful bladder infections account for the bulk of these visits. If you think that you are getting a bladder infection, drink lots of cranberry juice, monitor your condition, and get help if your symptoms persist. When I developed sudden urinary retention after surgery about ten years ago, I though that I would explode! My sympathies go to anyone who might have a similar experience.

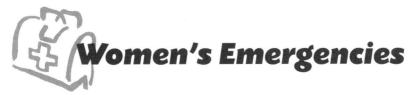

Women's Emergencies

Gynecological Emergencies

What They Are

Women's emergencies usually fall into two basic categories, those involving pregnancy and abnormal inflammation or bleeding in the reproductive organs. The early diagnosis of gynecological emergencies can be difficult because of the complex anatomy involved and because many of the symptoms are shared with other ailments.

Vaginal Bleeding

During normal menstruation, blood loss is between 30 to 60 ccs. (requiring one to three tampons for absorption). Women may also experience a consistent pattern of mild cramping at certain points of the menstrual cycle over the course of their lives. Vaginal bleeding becomes a medical emergency when the volume of blood, the duration of the bleeding, the time of the month when bleeding occurs and other symptoms (cramping, vomiting, abdominal pain, and clotting) differ from the patient's usual menstrual pattern. Since normal menstrual bleeding doesn't clot, heavy or rapid bleeding and the presence of clots may indicate abnormalities including fibroid tumors, endocrine imbalances, or cancer of the uterus or cervix. Both birth control pills and estrogen replacement therapy can also cause abnormal or heavy bleeding. Post-menopausal bleeding always requires evaluation.

Fibroid Tumors

About twenty-five percent of women have fibroid tumors—abnormal muscle growths in the womb. After years of unnoticed enlargement, fibroid tumors can bleed excessively, but few hemorrhage enough to require urgent care. Gynecologists can often feel fibroid tumors during pelvic examinations.

Ovarian Cysts
Abnormal ovulation can cause ovarian cysts, small growths on the surface of the ovary that may swell and rupture. A bursting ovarian cyst immediately causes severe discomfort. In contrast, ovarian cancer grows slowly and silently making detection difficult.

Tubal Pregnancies
Abdominal or pelvic pain without vaginal bleeding can indicate a tubal (ectopic) pregnancy. A tubal pregnancy occurs when a fertilized egg is implanted in a Fallopian tube, not in the uterine wall. The surrounding tissues can't support fetal development. Intense pain and nausea ensue. When the fetus dies and uterine bleeding is heavy, the patient's blood pressure may suddenly drop. Tubal pregnancy occurs in about two percent of all pregnancies. It is the most lethal gynecological emergency because blood may enter and irritate the abdominal cavity.

Other causes of heavy menstrual bleeding and/or pelvic pain include:
- Benign polyps of the cervix or uterus—the excessive growth of normal tissue.
- Pelvic inflammatory disease of the female reproductive organs (PID)—is usually a sexually transmitted disease (gonorrhea or chlamydia) affecting the Fallopian tubes, uterus, or an ovary. It often forms abscesses that rupture, leading to bacterial peritonitis.
- Endometriosis—The implanting of normal uterine tissue in abnormal areas of the pelvis or abdomen. Endometriosis is found in five to ten percent of women and is thought to be due to retrograde menstruation (menstruation that flows in the wrong direction). It causes cyclical discomfort that will be continuous if scarring occurs.

Women's Emergencies

What To Look For
- Heavy or rapid vaginal bleeding.
- Sudden or severe pelvic or abdominal pain.
- Nausea, vomiting.
- Fever, vaginal discharge, lower abdominal pain (PID or pelvic abscess).
- Fatigue, nausea, and loss of appetite (could indicate the spread of uterine or cervical cancer).
- Dizziness, light-headedness, anxiety, or fainting (may be signs of unstable blood pressure).
- Shoulder pain may be due to blood irritating the inner abdominal membranes and the lower diaphragm surface (possibly indicating a tubal pregnancy).

What To Do
- Call 911 immediately.
- Have the patient rest comfortably, preferably lying down with her knees elevated to avoid dizziness, faintness, or collapse.
- Gynecological emergencies are always emotionally draining so patients will need both cardiovascular and psychological support.

What Not To Do
- Don't leave patients unattended after calling 911.
- Don't allow patients to eat, drink, or take over-the-counter medications. For example, aspirin could thin the blood and worsen hemorrhaging, and Tylenol® could mask characteristic painful symptoms.
- Don't touch the abdomen. It could lead to nausea, vomiting, or circulatory collapse if pressure causes an ovarian cyst, tubal pregnancy, or pelvic abscess to rupture.

Typical Treatment
Emergency personnel will assess the severity of the patient's condition by checking

her vital signs. Their primary concern is stabilizing her blood pressure and tissue oxygenation.

Laboratory testing will determine if a patient is pregnant. If she has lost substantial amounts of blood she will be given intravenous fluids, nasal oxygen, and perhaps transfusions. Her pelvic organs will be examined for signs of bleeding, infection, uterine fibroids, ovarian masses, and cancer.

A patient with a tubal pregnancy will receive immediate surgery if she has low blood pressure, a fast heart rate, and a low blood count. Some younger patients may be candidates for limited surgery to remove only the affected portion of the Fallopian tube while others might be injected with methotrexate, which causes a tubal abortion.

Often, a pelvic sonogram can identify tubal pregnancy, fibroid tumors, ovarian cysts/abscesses, endometriosis, and some cancers. If found, a hysteroscopy (a uterus examination using a fiber-optic camera) or a biopsy may be needed.

Women over thirty-five who have abnormal vaginal bleeding may be treated as outpatients if their vital signs and test results are normal.

Gynecological emergencies not due to pregnancy must be evaluated for irritation or infection of the abdominal cavity (peritonitis). If blood has entered the abdomen, immediate exploratory surgery will be necessary.

Vaginal bleeding due to fibroid tumors, cancer, or infection will be treated when the underlying condition is diagnosed.

PID is treated with oral or intravenous antibiotics. Severe cases are admitted for hospitalization to prevent complications such as tubal pregnancy and infertility.

Many subtypes of menstrual bleeding respond to estrogen therapy, birth control pills, or anti-inflammatory medications such as ibuprofen and Naprosyn®.

Follow-up Care

The length of hospitalization depends on the type of emergency and the extent of bleeding, infection, or secondary complications including peritonitis. The patient should be examined by her gynecologist a few days after being discharged from the hospital.

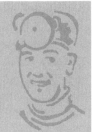

Dr. Fischer Says

Regular gynecologic checkups are essential. Often, they can prevent the onset of serious emergencies. Many PID cases are undiagnosed and can lead to tubal pregnancies and infertility. Patients who suspect PID should get prompt treatment and counseling as should their partners. Postmenopausal bleeding and abdominal pain during menstruation are always abnormal, so immediately see your doctor.

Obstetric Disorders

What They Are

During pregnancy, women can develop a number of conditions that can endanger both the fetus and themselves. Some of these conditions are:

High Blood Pressure

Women who normally don't have high blood pressure often develop elevated readings during the second 20 weeks of pregnancy. Those whose readings exceed 140/90 must be monitored throughout the full term of their pregnancies. Hypertensive women should follow a low salt diet, monitor their weight gain, and may have to take blood pressure medication.

Preeclampsia

Some women will accumulate excessive tissue fluid and their hands, face, and legs will swell. If women who retain fluid also have protein in their urine, it means that they have preeclampsia. This condition can cause frontal headaches, blurred vision, upper right abdominal pain, and overactive reflexes. If untreated, preeclampsia can turn into *eclampsia*, an emergency characterized by convulsions that violently shake the entire body, causing loss of consciousness, and danger to the fetus.

Blood Clots

Pregnant women may develop clots in the deep veins of their legs. Clots are formed because the pregnant uterus slows the return of blood through the leg veins and because chemicals that promote clotting increase. Clots may break free and travel to the lungs (pulmonary emboli), an emergency that can be fatal.

Vaginal Bleeding

In the first twenty weeks of pregnancy, bleeding usually indicates spontaneous termination of pregnancy, which may be accompanied by pain, cramping, tenderness, and fever.

Placenta Previa and Placental Abruption

Bleeding in the second twenty weeks is usually due to placenta previa or placental abruption.

Placenta previa occurs when the developing fetus pushes an abnormally low-lying placenta off the uterine wall causing severe shock, fainting, paleness, and an extremely weak pulse. Patients develop bright red bleeding that may be painless. At first, bleeding is slight, but it recurs and worsens over several days.

Placental abruption occurs when the placenta prematurely separates from its usual location on the upper uterine wall. Usually, it entails profuse, dark, and often clotted vaginal bleeding causing severe shock, fainting, paleness, and an extremely weak pulse. However, blood can be trapped between the placenta and the uterine wall giving no obvious signs of bleeding. Women may report abdominal, pelvic, or back pain. High blood pressure and physical trauma may cause placental abruption.

Cancer, Polyps, Kidney Infections, and Other Conditions
All of these conditions can cause vaginal bleeding and threaten the fetus.

What To Look For
- Fluid retention and swollen hands, face, and legs throughout the day (*preeclampsia*).
- Frontal headaches, blurred vision, upper right abdominal pain, and overactive reflexes (*preeclampsia*).
- Uncontrollable shaking throughout the body, followed by stiffness, confusion, and disorientation (*eclampsia*).
- Pain, swelling, and warmth in either calf (*deep-vein thrombosis*).
- Vaginal bleeding with cramping, tenderness, or fever in the first twenty weeks of pregnancy (*spontaneous termination of pregnancy*).
- Paleness, cold and clammy skin, and agitation (*excessive blood loss*).
- Painless, bright red vaginal bleeding in the second twenty weeks of pregnancy (*placenta previa*).
- Vaginal bleeding that is heavy, dark, and clotted. Shock, fainting, paleness, and an extremely weak pulse in the second twenty weeks of pregnancy (*placental abruption*).
- Uterine contractions and gush of fluid before the expected date of delivery (*premature rupture of membranes*).
- Abdominal pain. While nausea and vomiting are common in pregnancy, abdominal pain is not and may indicate a potential emergency.

What To Do
- If a pregnant woman begins to shake uncontrollably over her entire body and then becomes stiff, confused, and disoriented, call 911 immediately. Assume that the patient has eclampsia if she has such seizures in the second half of pregnancy.
- Patients with swelling, pain, and warmness in either calf may have a blood clot. Call 911 at once and keep them sitting or lying down.

- When patients bleed vaginally and have cramps, tenderness, fever, paleness, coldness, clammy skin, or agitation (spontaneous termination of pregnancy, placental injury), call 911 immediately.

What Not To Do

- Don't let patients with leg pain stand, walk, or be active. They may have blood clots in their legs that could dislodge, travel to the lungs, and impair the circulation of oxygen to vital organs.

Typical Treatment

The first step in treating obstetric emergencies is checking and stabilizing the patient's circulation and blood flow. A sonogram will then determine the age and the condition of the fetus. Lab tests will reveal the extent of blood loss and the approximate duration of the pregnancy.

Eclampsia

Patients with blood pressure over 140/90, and those with lower readings who exhibit any suspicious signs or symptoms, will be hospitalized. Preeclampsia requires bed rest, monitoring blood pressure, and frequent obstetrician visits. Seizures affecting eclampsia patients will be controlled with intravenous magnesium sulfate or antiepileptic and blood pressure medication. When the patient's condition has stabilized, a decision will be made whether to surgically deliver the child (by Caesarian section) or allow the pregnancy to continue. It may be safer to care for a premature newborn in the neonatal intensive care unit than to let it remain in the mother's uterus where it could be injured if the mother has convulsions or circulatory problems. Since eclampsia is triggered by the release of hormones during pregnancy, it resolves after delivery.

Phlebitis

Patients with blood clots will be hospitalized and given intravenous blood thinners. Specialized radiological testing such as Doppler sonography and venography will show whether clots have dissolved and normal blood flow has been restored. If there is risk of hemorrhage or the mother's death, a decision must be made at the thirty-fourth to thirty-sixth week of gestation whether or not to deliver the baby (and transfer it to a neonatal intensive care unit).

Placental Injury

Placental abruption and bleeding placenta previa patients will immediately receive intravenous fluids and oxygen. They will be rushed to the delivery room for Caesarean delivery. Newborns are then monitored in the intensive care unit and the mothers will remain hospitalized until their conditions stabilize.

Premature Labor/ Rupture of Membranes

New medications (tocolytics) can inhibit labor contractions for several days and provide time for the mother to get to a facility with a neonatal ICU. Among the drugs available are terbutaline, magnesium sulfate, nifedipine, and steroids. They may be used only if the fetus is between twenty-four to thirty-four weeks of gestation.

Follow-up Care

Obstetric emergencies are extremely serious and often require a week or more of postpartum hospitalization. Massive bleeding and pelvic infections are two emergencies that commonly occur during the postpartum period, requiring observation in the hospital for several days after delivery.

Dr. Fischer Says

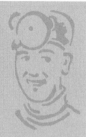

Monitor all pregnancies whether they are high-risk or not to reduce the risk of unhappy complications. Remember—obstetric problems involve both the lives of expectant mothers and their children. Since many of the same problems can recur during subsequent pregnancies, mothers should get frequent checkups to monitor their conditions when they become pregnant again.

Procedures

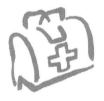

How To Take a Pulse

Our heart pumps blood through the body in a regular rhythm or cadence. At certain points on the body, we can feel that rhythm or pulse and measure its beat. If we feel a pulse, we know that the heart is beating, which means that the patient is alive. If we count the number of beats, we can calculate the rate or strength with which the heart is beating.

Although the pulse can be felt at a number of locations, the easiest places for most people to access are the wrist and carotid artery in the neck. Finding a pulse can be frustrating, especially the first few times you try. So practice on yourself and/or on your family so you can find a pulse quickly in a medical emergency.

In medical emergencies, don't bother to calculate the patient's pulse rate. Simply try to find the patient's pulse and whether it's beating strongly, weakly, or not at all. If the patient isn't breathing and you can't find a pulse within ten seconds, begin CPR.

To take a pulse:

On the Wrist
Place the pads of your index and middle fingers on the groove on the inner side of the patient's wrist just up the arm from the bone at the base of the thumb (about one inch up from the place where the hand meets the wrist). Move your fingers lightly until you feel intermittent pulsations.

How To Take a Pulse

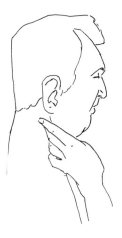

On the Neck

Lift the chin slightly and lightly run the pads of your three middle fingers along the outer edge of the windpipe under the patient's jaw and alongside the Adam's apple. Keep moving your fingers until you feel intermittent pulsations.

Figuring the Pulse Rate

Once you have found the pulse, press gently, and keep your fingers in place. Then count the number of pulsations you feel in a ten-second period. Multiply the number of pulsations by six to get the patient's pulse rate per minute.

How To Give CPR

Cardiopulmonary rescuscitation (CPR) is used to try to revive patients who are not breathing and/or have no heartbeat (pulse). It is used when patients have:

- Collapsed and are unresponsive.
- Stopped breathing.
- No pulse.
- Blue lips, fingers, or face.

What to Do

1. Check the patient's responsiveness:
   - Gently tap the patient's shoulder and ask, "Are you OK?" Speak loudly and repeat several times, if necessary. Patients having massive heart attacks, drug overdoses, or serious head injuries usually won't respond, but those who are simply intoxicated, fainting, or asleep will generally answer promptly.
   - Check the patient's breathing. Remove or open clothing to see if the chest rises and falls. Place your ear by the nose and mouth to hear or feel the passage of air. If, after several seconds, there is no chest movement, proceed as if the patient is unresponsive.

2. Call 911, even if you have to leave the patient alone. If you are not alone, someone should stay

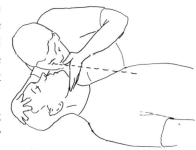

with the patient while another person calls 911. Time is of the essence: the sooner trained emergency personnel arrive and begin advanced cardiac life support, the greater the chances of survival.

3. Immediately place the patient flat on his/her back and elevate the legs slightly to improve circulation to the vital organs. However, *don't move patients with suspected neck injuries!*

4. Tilt the head back slightly to establish an airway. If necessary, place your hand under the patient's neck to lift his/her chin upward and forward to fully open the mouth. This will also prevent the tongue from blocking airflow to and from the lungs.

5. Administer *mouth-to-mouth resuscitation*:
   - Take a deep breath.
   - Pinch the patient's nostrils.
   - Place your mouth directly on the patient's mouth.
   - Slowly exhale fully into the patient's mouth filling up his/her lungs.
   - Repeat one more time.
   - Check that the patient's chest rises and falls between breaths (to see that the air goes in).
   - If the lungs fail to expand, the patient may have an upper airway obstruction. If so, see p. 178.
   - Observe the patient's chest and put your ear to their mouth and nose to determine if the victim is breathing on his/her own.

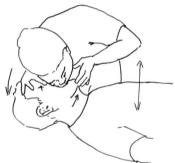

6. Place two fingers (other than your thumb) on the artery that runs to the side of the Adam's apple and feel for a pulse. If you find a pulse, some functions (breath-

ing and heart) may have been restored, but the patient's blood pressure and normal circulation may still be impaired.

7. If you don't feel a pulse after ten seconds, immediately begin chest compressions. Kneel next to the patient with your knees by the victim's shoulder and upper arm.

For Adults

Place the heel of one hand two inches above the center of the lower tip of the patient's breastbone and the other hand directly on top of it, so that one hand covers most of the other. Move your torso directly over the patient so your arms point straight down towards his chest. With your elbows straight and locked, press directly down on the breastbone *one and one half to two inches*. Apply pressure with the heel of your lower palm, not with your fingers, which could fracture a rib. Hold each compression for about one second.

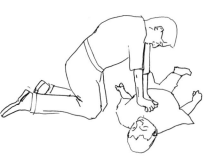

For Children
- Press with the heel of *one* hand only to compress the breastbone about *one inch*.
- Place the other hand on the forehead to keep the airway open.

For Infants
- Use *two fingers* of one hand to compress the breastbone about *a half-inch*.
- Continue CPR without stopping until emergency help arrives.

One-Rescuer CPR
- If alone, compress the chest fifteen times.
- Give two mouth-to-mouth respirations.
- Continue the fifteen-to-two ratio until 911 arrives.

- Periodically check to see if the patient's heart has begun to beat (feel the neck artery) or there is spontaneous breathing. After a few seconds, if there is neither breathing nor a heartbeat, resume CPR.

Two-Rescuer CPR

- One person should apply chest compressions while the other gives mouth-to-mouth resuscitation.
- Give five chest compressions followed immediately by one mouth-to-mouth respiration.
- Continue this five-to-one pattern until emergency personnel arrive.
- To avoid fatigue, rescuers should rotate duties and, in the interval when they switch, check if the patient is breathing or has a heartbeat.
- If the patient begins breathing and his/her heart begins beating, place the patient on his/her side.

What Not To Do

- Don't move patients who may have neck injuries.
- In giving chest compressions, don't apply pressure with your fingers because the force could break a rib. Instead, press straight downward with the heel of your hand.

Typical Treatment

When emergency personnel arrive, they will continue CPR. They'll also give advanced cardiac life support—treatment that improves oxygenation, treats potentially lethal heart rhythm disturbances, and hopefully restores blood pressure and circulation.

Survivors of cardiopulmonary arrest will be hospitalized and monitored in an intensive care unit. Dangerous heart rhythms often occur during the first twenty-four hours; these may require immediate administration of intravenous medication or electrical defibrillation. The length of a patient's hospitalization will depend on the gravity of each individual case.

Dr. Fischer Says

When you call 911, help won't arrive for at least several minutes so your ability to perform CPR may keep the patient alive. Learn CPR. The American Red Cross provides excellent CPR courses that teach the physical skills needed to perform this often lifesaving therapy.

There is no evidence of AIDS being contracted through mouth-to-mouth resuscitation. Experts believe that saliva protects caretakers so giving CPR should never be delayed to look for plastic shields, tissues, or other forms of protection. 911 personnel use specialized ventilation equipment.

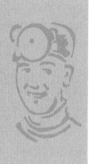

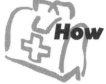

How To Dislodge an Obstruction From the Throat

What To Look For
- Coughing, gasping for air, and/or clutching the throat.
- Fast and deep breathing.
- Change in the patient's voice (partial obstruction).
- Inability to talk (total obstruction).
- Wheezing (from trying to force air around the trapped object).
- Blue fingers, lips, and face.
- Collapse, unconsciousness.

What To Do
Conscious Patients
- Keep patients erect, with their heads leaning slightly forward. Call 911 immediately if they can talk, cough, and breathe without assistance. Allow alert patients with partial obstruction to try to clear the blockage on their own.
- If patients can't talk, breathe or cough: perform abdominal thrusts *(Heimlich Maneuver)* as follows:
1. Stand directly behind the patient.
2. Wrap your arms around the patient's waist.
3. Clasp your hands above the navel, under the ribcage, so your thumb is pressing against the patient's abdomen. Be sure your hands are several inches below the lower tip of the patient's breastbone.

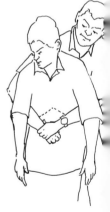

How To Dislodge an Obstruction From the Throat

4. Pull inwards and upwards five (5) times in succession.
5. After each cycle of five (5) thrusts, gently sweep the patient's mouth with your finger to see if the object has popped out and can be removed.
6. Repeat the cycle of five (5) abdominal thrusts until the object dislodges, the person becomes unconscious or collapses, or emergency personnel arrive.

Unconscious Patients

- Call 911 immediately.
- If a patient inhaled vomit, turn the victim on his/her stomach with the head as far down as possible. This should move the tongue forward and allow gastric contents to empty out of the mouth, not into the lungs.

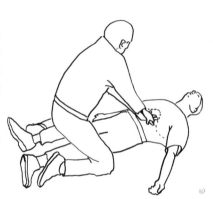

1. Turn the patient on his/her back and kneel along side his/her hips facing the patient's head.
2. Deliver five (5) abdominal thrusts (Heimlich Maneuver) by:
   A. Pressing the heels of your hands above the patient's navel, several inches under the ribcage. Be sure your hands are below the lower tip of the breastbone.
   B. Push inwards toward the shoulders five (5) times in succession.
   C. After each cycle, gently sweep the patient's mouth with your finger to see if the object has popped out and can be removed.
   D. Repeating the cycle of five (5) abdominal thrusts and checking the patient's mouth until the obstructing object is dislodged, the person becomes conscious, or emergency personnel arrive.

How To Dislodge an Obstruction From the Throat

Choking Infants
- Place the child on his/her back.
- Place two (2) fingers between the navel and rib cage and compress downwards and towards the shoulders several times.
- Check the child's mouth to see if the object has popped out and can be removed. Proceed cautiously because it is easy to push objects back into the trachea. Continue until help arrives.

If You Are Choking
- Stand facing the back of a chair or over a railing.
- Place your fist between your navel and rib cage.
- Lean downward quickly into the chair or railing so that your fist presses into the abdomen and upward toward the shoulders.
- Repeat until you feel the object pop out, you can breathe normally, or until help arrives.

How To Stop Bleeding Wounds

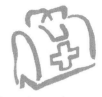

Most bleeding from wounds can be stopped when you apply pressure directly on the wound. Use tourniquets only if direct pressure did not stop the flow. Tourniquets can cut off circulation—so use them only when direct pressure fails.

What To Do

- Call 911 immediately.
- Remove or cut the patient's clothing to find the wound.
- Press directly on the wound with clean dressing, absorbent pads, bandages, gauze, or cloth.
- Keep pressing until the bleeding stops.
- Do not remove the dressing even after it becomes saturated with blood. If necessary, place other dressings over saturated ones.
- For injuries to limbs, lift the wounded arm or leg until it is above heart level. Don't elevate a broken limb.
- If the bleeding does not stop, try to find the pressure point (i.e. an artery) with the hand that is not applying direct pressure on the wound and apply pressure on the pressure point.
- *Tourniquets.* Wrap a belt, rope, or piece of fabric between the patient's heart and the wound. Wrap it loosely enough to place a stick or rigid object under the tourniquet next to the skin. Turn the stick to tighten the tourniquet. Apply a light touch and tighten the tourniquet only enough to stop the blood flow to the wound; don't strangle the limb. Don't loosen the tourniquet until emergency rescue workers arrive.

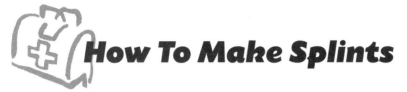# *How To Make Splints*

Stabilize broken or dislocated bones, sprains, strains, and severe cuts by applying splints to limit movement and to prevent further injury. Immobilizing injuries prevents fractured bones from moving and damaging nerves and blood vessels. Splints also help reduce pain and limit shock.

To make a splint, use any material at hand that can support the damaged area: wood, plastic, metal, cardboard, magazines, books, fabric, and even sheets of paper.

What To Do

- Loosen or remove any tight or constricting clothing.
- Place the splint material directly next to or under the injured area. Splint both joints around an injured limb. For a forearm injury, splint the arm beyond both the wrist and the elbow to limit movement in these joints.
- Remove jewelry that could cut off circulation when the injured area swells. Put the jewelry in the patient's pocket.
- Cushion the splint with soft padding. You may have to cut up some of your or the patient's clothing.
- Try not to move injured limbs. If this is impossible, gently lift the injured limb with both hands in one motion without disturbing any broken bones. Then carefully place the injured limb on the splint.
- Secure the splint by tying rope, string, a belt, ties or strips of fabric around the injured limb. Don't cut off circulation and try not to wrap or knot the fasteners directly over the site of the injury.

How To Make Splints

- Put ice in a towel or cloth directly over a fracture, but don't put ice directly on the break.
- Elevate the limb above heart level to minimize swelling.
- Regularly check the splint to make sure that swelling hasn't cut off circulation. If so, loosen it.

What Not To Do

- Don't move a patient if you even remotely suspect a broken neck.
- Don't try to align or set a broken bone.
- Don't push protruding bones back under the skin.

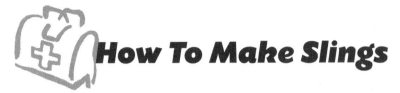# *How To Make Slings*

Essentially, a sling is a bandage draped around a patient's neck to immobilize, support, and protect an injured arm from further damage. Triangular cloths or bandages and bandannas make ideal slings, but when they are not available you will have to improvise by using, and often cutting up, clothing and other nonstretch material. In a pinch, even panty hose can work.

What To Do

1. Use a triangular cloth, bandage, or any nonstretch material that can be tied around the patient's neck to hold the injured arm (a tie, belt, pieces of clothing).
2. Put one corner of the triangle around the patient's neck on the side opposite the injury. Then place another corner so that it is pointing downward and the third by the patient's elbow.
3. Gently bend the injured arm so that the patient's hand is slightly higher than his/her elbow and across his/her chest.
4. Place the injured arm in the broadest part of the triangle and adjust it so that the support does not press directly on the injured area.
5. Tie the corner around the patient's neck with the corner that originally pointed downward so that the patient's arm is cushioned at slightly less than a ninety-degree angle (hand higher than elbow).
6. Tie the sling with a knot at the side of the patient's neck opposite the injury and cushion the knot with cloth or a handkerchief so that it doesn't dig into the patient.

How To Make Slings

7. Secure the patient's injured arm to his/her torso by wrapping a bandage, rope, or fabric over the injured arm, around the back and under the uninjured arm.

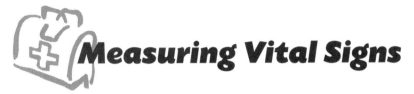

Measuring Vital Signs

Measuring a patient's vital signs provides invaluable information on the patient's condition. In medical emergencies, ambulance and emergency care workers will check a patient's vital signs while they ask some basic questions, before they begin any tests or treatments. The vital signs will help them determine the nature of the patient's problem.

The vital signs that are measured are:
- Temperature.
- Heart rate.
- Breathing rate.
- Blood pressure.

Any disorder that depletes the body of water, tissue fluid, or blood lowers blood pressure and triggers an accelerated heart rate. When body temperature is raised just one degree, the pulse increases by ten beats per minute.

Blood circulates oxygen throughout our bodies and must be chemically balanced for us to function properly. Diseases that increase the amount of dissolved acid in the blood produce a state of acidosis (kidney failure, asthma) and cause the patient's respiratory rate to rise (over the normal 18 breaths per minute). Illnesses that slow the heart (certain rhythm disturbances) or breathing (opiate overdoses) can abruptly change the acid/base balance and stop the heart.

Shock
Patients go "into shock" when their blood circulation becomes critically poor and

jeopardizes vital organs. When cells in the heart, brain, and kidneys are deprived of oxygen for several minutes they die. Patients in shock usually have very low blood pressure, often under 80/50. Shock can be brought on by severe fluid and/or blood loss from burns or an injured artery, by impaired pumping of blood during a heart attack, as well as by blood-borne infections, severe allergic reactions, and cervical (neck) spinal cord injuries.

Mental Status

In the ER, the staff will usually check a "fifth vital sign:" the patient's mental status. Many medical emergencies can change a patient's levels of orientation, awareness, and thinking. Reflexes can dramatically change and the patient may be unable to move or communicate. A wide variety of conditions can alter a patient's mental status including injury (bleeding into the brain), infections (encephalitis, meningitis), and intoxication from alcohol and/or drugs. Examples of heightened forms of altered mental status are agitation, delirium, and dementia. Stupor and coma are states of depressed or absent brain activity. A patient's mental status may change during the course of his/her observation (for either better or worse), which may provide information that will help in diagnosing the source of the problem.

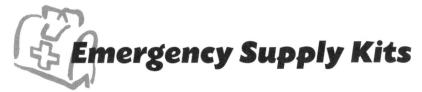 Emergency Supply Kits

Create an emergency supply kit for your home, place of business, vehicle, or boat. Use the list below as a guideline to stock a kit that meets your needs. In creating a kit, consider factors such as where you live and your distance from an emergency care center. Also factor in who might need first aid care and whether they suffer from any particular medical conditions.

You probably already have many of the items listed below, so just fill in the gaps because you never know when you may need them. Check the expiration dates on all your supplies. Many first aid supplies should be replaced after one year.

A number of vendors sell prepackaged, emergency supply kits, including the American Red Cross, which sells a number of kits. Many come in durable, weatherproof containers and by buying from the Red Cross you are supporting a worthy organization.

Supply Kit Checklist

___ Disposable protective gloves
___ Flashlight and extra batteries
___ EpiPen®
___ Snakebite extractor
___ Knife
___ Scissors and/or shears
___ Tweezers
___ Thermometer

___ Blankets
___ Water. 1 gallon per person per day for 3 days
___ Plastic bags, assorted sizes
___ Adhesive bandages, in assorted sizes
___ Adhesive tape, 1/2 or 1 inch
___ Butterfly closures
___ Hypoallergic tape

Emergency Supply Kits

- ___ Waterproof tape
- ___ Triangular bandages
- ___ Safety pins, medium size
- ___ Duct tape
- ___ Mole skin or Molefoam
- ___ Sterile cotton balls
- ___ Gauze pads, 2 x 2, 2 x 3 and 4 x 4
- ___ Gauze rolls
- ___ Nonstick pads, 2 by 3 and 3 by 4
- ___ Sanitary napkins
- ___ Tissues
- ___ Alcohol cleansing pads
- ___ Antiseptic wipes
- ___ Cotton swabs
- ___ Disposable instant-activating cold packs
- ___ Aspirin or nonaspirin pain relievers
- ___ Antacid
- ___ Motion sickness pills
- ___ Antidiarrheal medicine
- ___ Benadryl® or anti-allergy pills (even if no one has been diagnosed with sting or food allergies)
- ___ Decongestant tablets or nasal spray
- ___ Ipecac syrup
- ___ Calamine lotion
- ___ Antiseptic lotion
- ___ Triple antibiotic ointment
- ___ Anti-itching ointment
- ___ Burn relief gel packs
- ___ Sunblock

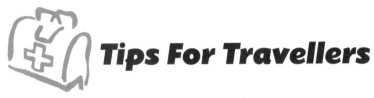

Tips For Travellers

How To Prepare For Medical Emergencies When You Are Away From Home

Whether you are out jogging near your home or traveling in a foreign country, it is a good idea to carry a card that has vital information about your health. This card should contain the following information, but you may want to add to it:

1. Your name, address, and the phone number where you are staying.
2. Name of a person to contact in an emergency.
3. Any medical problems or allergies you may have, including allergy to medication.
4. List of medications you are taking.
5. Your physician's name, address, and phone number.

If you have a cell phone, carry it with you. It could be your lifeline in an emergency.

If you have a potentially serious health problem and are staying at a hotel or someone's home, ask where the nearest hospital is. Find out what the procedure is to get you there if the need arises.

For Travel Abroad

1. Before you leave, find out what immunizations you need. Contact the U.S. Centers for Disease Control and Prevention's International Traveler's Hotline at 877-394-8747, www.cdc.gov/travel, or the International Association for Medical Assistance to Travelers at www.iamat.org. Both provide information on vaccinations, outbreaks in areas where you plan to travel, and much more.

2. Schedule immunizations in advance. Get your shots early because they may take time to take effect and certain countries will bar your entry if your immunization

is not yet effective. In addition, some immunizations may entail a series of inoculations and you may have adverse reactions that could delay the process. Finally, personal physicians are usually not equipped to give all immunizations and you may end up having to go to a special health center, which could take time to locate, schedule, and visit.

3. See your personal physician for a physical examination, to get all necessary booster shots, and to update your prescriptions. Get a written copy of all your prescriptions and have your doctor write their generic names so that they can be easily understood and filled abroad.

4. Have your physician complete a personal medical record for you to carry during your travels. The record should list your chronic medical conditions, recent disorders, allergies, and blood type. Also carry your physician's name, address, and phone number.

5. Carry your prescription medicines in their original containers with their original labels or carry copies of your prescriptions signed by your doctor. This can facilitate getting refills and avoid hassles with customs officials.

6. Join the International Association for Medical Travelers (IAMAT) (membership is free). In addition to providing information on international immunizations requirements, IAMAT publishes a listing of doctors in 125 countries who speak English. Also check out the U.S. Department of State Bureau of Consular affairs (http://travel.state.gov) for travel health information, travel warnings, help for Americans abroad, and lists of doctors, hospitals, and lawyers abroad.

7. Check your health care insurance to see if it covers the treatment of medical emergencies abroad. Many do not and others have limitations. *Medicare does not cover medical treatment received abroad* (except for hospitals in Canadian and Mexican border towns).

Tips For Travellers

8. If your health care insurance does not cover medical emergencies abroad, purchase a supplemental travel health insurance policy or an emergency assistance policy through your travel agent, your insurance agent, or the American Automobile Association. Make sure that the policy covers medical evacuation, which can be enormously expensive. Most companies that cover medical emergencies abroad provide twenty-four hour telephone-operator service and will direct you to doctors and hospitals. Some will send checks to pay your emergency medical costs, which can be important since many foreign medical providers won't bill your insurance carrier and insist on payment on the spot.

9. Consider joining MedJet Assistance, a pre-paid subscription service that will fly you from any place in the world to the hospital of your choice. If you are hospitalized, MedJet, which operates 365 days per year, will evacuate you in specially equipped jets staffed by medical teams. The yearly fee is $175 per person or $275 for families. (www.medjetassistance.com, 800-963-3538).

10. Leave a copy of your itinerary with a reliable friend or member of your family. Include in your itinerary all your air, sea, and ground travel departure and arrival times; all flight, ship, and train numbers; the name, address, and phone number of your hotels or places where you will be staying, and your doctor's name and phone number.

11. Should you incur any medical problems abroad, make an appointment upon your return to see and discuss it with your physician or an appropriate specialist. Parasites and exposures to exotic illnesses are an inherent risk of foreign travel. In addition, airplanes are closed compartments that act as incubators for airborne illness.

Poison Center Locations in the United States

American Association of Poison Control Centers
U.S. Poison Control Center Members
December, 2001

ALABAMA
Alabama Poison Center
2503 Phoenix Drive
Tuscaloosa, AL 35405
Emergency Phone: (800) 222-1222

Regional Poison Control Center
Children's Hospital
1600 7th Avenue South
Birmingham, AL 35233
Emergency Phone: (800) 222-1222

ARIZONA
Arizona Poison & Drug Info Center
Arizona Health Sciences Center, Room 1156
1501 North Campbell Avenue
Tucson, AZ 85724
Emergency Phone: (800) 222-1222

Samaritan Regional Poison Center
Good Samaritan Regional Medical Center
1111 E. McDowell--Ancillary 1
Phoenix, AZ 85006
Emergency Phone: (800) 222-1222

ARKANSAS
Arkansas Poison & Drug Information Center
College of Pharmacy
University of Arkansas for Medical Sciences
4301 W. Markham, Mail Slot 522
Little Rock, AR 72205
Emergency Phone: (800) 222-1222

CALIFORNIA
California Poison Control System -
Fresno/Madera Division
Valley Children's Hospital
9300 Valley Children's Place, MB 15
Madera, CA 93638-8762
Emergency Phone: (800) 222-1222

Poison Center Locations in the United States

California Poison Control System - Sacramento Division
UC Davis Medical Center
2315 Stockton Boulevard
Sacramento, CA 95817
Emergency Phone: (800) 222-1222

California Poison Control System - San Diego Division
University of California, San Diego, Medical Center
200 West Arbor Drive
San Diego, CA 92103-8925
Emergency Phone: (800) 222-1222

California Poison Control System - San Francisco Division
UCSF Box 1369
1001 Potrero Avenue, Room 1E86
San Francisco, CA 94143-1369
Emergency Phone: (800) 222-1222

COLORADO
Rocky Mountain Poison & Drug Ctr
1010 Yosemite Street, Suite 200
Denver, CO 80230-6800
Emergency Phone: (800) 222-1222

CONNECTICUT
Connecticut Poison Control Center
University of Connecticut Health Center
263 Farmington Avenue
Farmington, CT 06030-5365
Emergency Phone: (800) 222-1222

DELAWARE
The Poison Control Center
3535 Market Street, Suite 985
Philadelphia, PA 19104-3309
Emergency Phone: (800) 222-1222

DISTRICT OF COLUMBIA
National Capital Poison Center
3201 New Mexico Avenue, Suite 310
Washington, DC 20016
Emergency Phone: (800) 222-1222

FLORIDA
Florida Poison Information Center - Jacksonville
655 West Eighth Street
Jacksonville, FL 32209
Emergency Phone: (800) 222-1222

Florida Poison Information Center - Miami
University of Miami, Dept of Pediatrics
Jackson Memorial Medical Center
P.O. Box 016960 (R-131)
Miami, FL 33101
Emergency Phone: (800) 222-1222

Poison Center Locations in the United States

Florida Poison Information Center - Tampa
Tampa General Hospital
P.O. Box 1289
Tampa, FL 33601
Emergency Phone: (800) 222-1222

GEORGIA
Georgia Poison Center
Hughes Spalding Children's Hospital
Grady Health System
80 Butler Street, SE
P.O. Box 26066
Atlanta, GA 30335-3801
Emergency Phone: (800) 222-1222

HAWAII
Hawaii Poison Center
Kapiolani Call Center Services
55 Merchant St., 27th Floor
Honolulu, HI 96813
Emergency Phone: (800) 222-1222

IDAHO
Rocky Mountain Poison & Drug Ctr
1010 Yosemite Street, Suite 200
Denver, CO 80230 6800
Emergency Phone: (800) 222-1222

ILLINOIS
Illinois Poison Center
222 S. Riverside Plaza, Suite 1900
Chicago, IL 60606
Emergency Phone: (800) 222-1222

INDIANA
Indiana Poison Center
Methodist Hospital
Clarian Health Partners
I-65 at 21st Street
Indianapolis, IN 46206-1367
Emergency Phone: (800) 222-1222

IOWA
Iowa Statewide Poison Control Center
St. Luke's Regional Medical Center
2720 Stone Park Boulevard
Sioux City, IA 51104
Emergency Phone: (800) 222-1222

KANSAS
Mid-America Poison Control Center
University of Kansas Medical Center
3901 Rainbow Blvd., Room B-400
Kansas City, KS 66160-7231
Emergency Phone: (800) 222-1222

KENTUCKY
Kentucky Regional Poison Center
Medical Towers South, Suite 572
234 East Gray Street
Louisville, KY 40202
Emergency Phone: (800) 222-1222

Poison Center Locations in the United States

LOUISIANA
Louisiana Drug and Poison Information Center
University of Louisiana at Monroe
College of Pharmacy, Sugar Hall
Monroe, LA 71209-6430
Emergency Phone: (800) 222-1222

MAINE
Maine Poison Center
Maine Medical Center
22 Bramhall Street
Portland, ME 04102
Emergency Phone: (800) 222-1222

MARYLAND
Maryland Poison Center
University of MD at Baltimore
School of Pharmacy
20 North Pine Street, PH 772
Baltimore, MD 21201
Emergency Phone: (800) 222-1222

National Capital Poison Center
3201 New Mexico Avenue, NW, Suite 310
Washington, DC 20016
Emergency Phone: (800) 222-1222

MASSACHUSETTS
Regional Center for Poison Control and
Prevention
Serving Massachusetts and Rhode Island
300 Longwood Avenue
Boston, MA 02115
Emergency Phone: (800) 222-1222

MICHIGAN
Children's Hospital of Michigan
Regional Poison Control Center
4160 John R Harper Professional Office Bldg,
Ste 616
Detroit, MI 48201
Emergency Phone: (800) 222-1222

DeVos Children's Hospital
Regional Poison Center
1300 Michigan, NE, Suite 203
Grand Rapids, MI 49503
Emergency Phone: (800) 222-1222

MINNESOTA
Hennepin Regional Poison Center
Hennepin County Medical Center
701 Park Avenue
Minneapolis, MN 55415
Emergency Phone: (800) 222-1222

Poison Center Locations in the United States

MISSISSIPPI
Mississippi Regional Poison Control Center
University of Mississippi Medical Center
2500 N. State Street
Jackson, MS 39216
Emergency Phone: (800) 222-1222

MISSOURI
Cardinal Glennon Children's Hospital
Regional Poison Center
1465 S. Grand Blvd.
St. Louis, MO 63104
Emergency Phone: (800) 222-1222

MONTANA
Rocky Mountain Poison & Drug Ctr
1010 Yosemite Street, Suite 200
Denver, CO 80230-6800
Emergency Phone: (800) 222-1222

NEBRASKA
The Poison Center
Children's Hospital
8200 Dodge Street
Omaha, NE 68114
Emergency Phone: (800) 222-1222

NEVADA
Oregon Poison Center
Oregon Health Sciences University
3181 SW Sam Jackson Park Road, CB550
Portland, OR 97201
Emergency Phone: (800) 222-1222

Rocky Mountain Poison & Drug Ctr
1010 Yosemite Street, Suite 200
Denver, CO 80230-6800
Emergency Phone: (800) 222-1222

NEW HAMPSHIRE
New Hampshire Poison Information Center
Dartmouth-Hitchcock Medical Center
One Medical Center Drive
Lebanon, NH 03756
Emergency Phone: (800) 222-1222

NEW JERSEY
New Jersey Poison Information and
Education System
201 Lyons Ave
Newark, NJ 07112
Emergency Phone: (800) 222-1222

NEW MEXICO
New Mexico Poison & Drug Information
Center
Health Science Center Library, Room 130
University of New Mexico
Albuquerque, NM 87131-1076
Emergency Phone: (800) 222-1222

NEW YORK
Central New York Poison Center
750 East Adams Street
Syracuse, NY 13210
Emergency Phone: (800) 222-1222

Poison Center Locations in the United States

Finger Lakes Regional Poison and Drug
Information Center
University of Rochester Medical Center
601 Elmwood Avenue, PO Box 321
Rochester, NY 14642
Emergency Phone: (800) 222-1222

Long Island Regional Poison and Drug
Information Center
Winthrop University Hospital
259 First Street
Mineola, NY 11501
Emergency Phone: (800) 222-1222

New York City Poison Control Center
NYC Bureau of Labs
455 First Avenue
Room 123, Box 81
New York, NY 10016
Emergency Phone: (800) 222-1222

Western New York Regional Poison Control
Center
Children's Hospital of Buffalo
219 Bryant Street
Buffalo, NY 14222
Emergency Phone: (800) 222-1222

NORTH CAROLINA
Carolinas Poison Center
Carolinas Medical Center
5000 Airport Center Parkway, Suite B
Charlotte, NC 28208
Emergency Phone: (800) 222-1222

NORTH DAKOTA
North Dakota Poison Information Center
Meritcare Medical Center
720 4th Street North
Fargo, ND 58122
Emergency Phone: (800) 222-1222

OHIO
Central Ohio Poison Center
700 Children's Drive, Room L032
Columbus, OH 43205
Emergency Phone: (800) 222-1222

Cincinnati Drug & Poison Information Center
Regional Poison Control System
3333 Burnet Avenue
Vernon Place - 3rd Floor
Cincinnati, OH 45229
Emergency Phone: (800) 222-1222

Greater Cleveland Poison Control Center
11100 Euclid Avenue
Cleveland, OH 44106-6010
Emergency Phone: (800) 222-1222

Poison Center Locations in the United States

OKLAHOMA
Oklahoma Poison Control Center
Children's Hospital at OU Medical Center
940 N.E. 13th Street, Room 3510
Oklahoma City, OK 73104
Emergency Phone: (800) 222-1222

OREGON
Oregon Poison Center
Oregon Health Sciences University
3181 SW Sam Jackson Park Road, CB550
Portland, OR 97201
Emergency Phone: (800) 222-1222

PENNSYLVANIA
Central Pennsylvania Poison Center
Pennsylvania State University
The Milton S. Hershey Medical Center
500 University Drive
MC H043, PO Box 850
Hershey, PA 17033-0850
Emergency Phone: (800) 222-1222

Pittsburgh Poison Center
Children's Hospital of Pittsburgh
3705 Fifth Avenue
Pittsburgh, PA 15213
Emergency Phone: (800) 222-1222

The Poison Control Center
3535 Market Street, Suite 985
Philadelphia, PA 19104-3309
Emergency Phone: (800) 222-1222

RHODE ISLAND
Regional Center for Poison Control and
Prevention
Serving Massachusetts and Rhode Island
300 Longwood Avenue
Boston, MA 02115
Emergency Phone: (800) 222-1222

SOUTH CAROLINA
Palmetto Poison Center
College of Pharmacy
University of South Carolina
Columbia, SC 29208
Emergency Phone: (800) 222-1222

SOUTH DAKOTA
Hennepin Regional Poison Center
Hennepin County Medical Center
701 Park Avenue
Minneapolis, MN 55415
Emergency Phone: (800) 222-1222

TENNESSEE
Middle Tennessee Poison Center
501 Oxford House
1161 21st Avenue South
Nashville, TN 37232-4632
Emergency Phone: (800) 222-1222

Poison Center Locations in the United States

Southern Poison Center
University of Tennessee
875 Monroe Avenue, Suite 104
Memphis, TN 38163
Emergency Phone: (800) 222-1222

TEXAS
Central Texas Poison Center
Scott and White Memorial Hospital
2401 South 31st Street
Temple, TX 76508
Emergency Phone: (800) 222-1222

North Texas Poison Center
Texas Poison Center Network
Parkland Health & Hospital System
5201 Harry Hines Blvd.
P.O. Box 35926
Dallas, TX 75235
Emergency Phone: (800) 222-1222

South Texas Poison Center
The Univ of Texas Health Science Ctr - San Antonio
Department of Surgery, Mail Code 7849
7703 Floyd Curl Drive
San Antonio, TX 78229-3900
Emergency Phone: (800) 222-1222

Southeast Texas Poison Center
The University of Texas Medical Branch
3.112 Trauma Building
Galveston, TX 77555-1175
Emergency Phone: (800) 222-1222

Texas Panhandle Poison Center
1501 S. Coulter
Amarillo, TX 79106
Emergency Phone: (800) 222-1222

West Texas Regional Poison Center
Thomason Hospital
4815 Alameda Avenue
El Paso, TX 79905
Emergency Phone: (800) 222-1222

UTAH
Utah Poison Control Center
410 Chipeta Way, Suite 230
Salt Lake City, UT 84108
Emergency Phone: (800) 222-1222

VERMONT
Maine Poison Center
Maine Medical Center
22 Bramhall Street
Portland, ME 04102
Emergency Phone: (800) 222-1222

Poison Center Locations in the United States

VIRGINIA
Blue Ridge Poison Center
University of Virginia Health System
PO Box 800774
Charlottesville, VA 22908-0774
Emergency Phone: (800) 222-1222

National Capital Poison Center
3201 New Mexico Avenue, NW, Suite 310
Washington, DC 20016
Emergency Phone: (800) 222-1222

Virginia Poison Center
Medical College of Virginia Hospitals
Virginia Commonwealth University
P.O. Box 980522
Richmond, VA 23298-0522
Emergency Phone: (800) 222-1222

WASHINGTON
Washington Poison Center
155 NE 100th Street, Suite 400
Seattle, WA 98125-8012
Emergency Phone: (800) 222-1222

WEST VIRGINIA
West Virginia Poison Center
3110 MacCorkle Ave, S.E.
Charleston, WV 25304
Emergency Phone: (800) 222-1222

WISCONSIN
Children's Hospital of Wisconsin Poison
Center
PO Box 1997, Mail Station 677A
Milwaukee, WI 53201-1997
Emergency Phone: (800) 222-1222

WYOMING
The Poison Center
Children's Hospital
8200 Dodge Street
Omaha, NE 68114
Emergency Phone: (800) 222-1222

Index

Index

Index

Index

Index